D0264874

The Prenatal Origin of Behavior

The Prenatal Origin of Behavior

by

Davenport Hooker, Ph.D., Sc.D.

Professor of Anatomy and Chairman of the Department
University of Pittsburgh School of Medicine

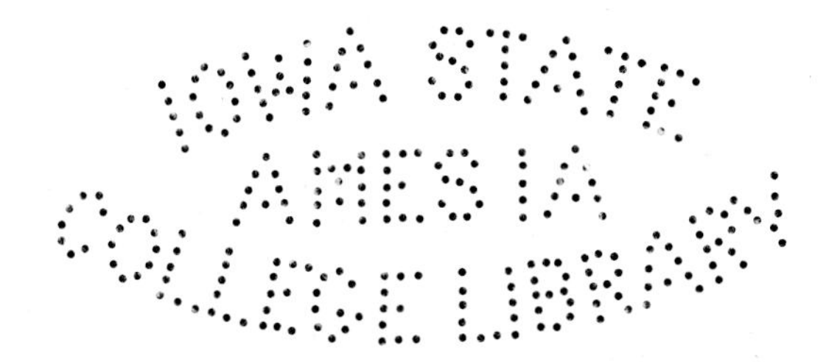

Porter Lectures, Series 18

University of Kansas Press, Lawrence, Kansas, 1952

Physiological and morphological studies on human prenatal development, publication no. 20. These studies have been aided by grants from the Penrose Fund of the American Philosophical Society, from the Carnegie Corporation of New York, from the University of Pittsburgh, and from the Sarah Mellon Scaife Foundation.

Preface

To be invited to fill the Porter Lectureship in Medicine is indeed an honor and one for which this lecturer is most grateful. Quite aside from my personal gratification at being invited to lecture on this foundation, I am especially pleased because of my long friendship with Dr. George Ellett Coghill, the founder in America of work on embryonic movements, who served the University of Kansas School of Medicine from 1913 to 1925. It has also been my privilege to know for a long time both Dr. Henry Carroll Tracy, his successor as Chairman of the Department at Kansas, and the present Chairman, Dr. Paul Gibbons Roofe.

I am indebted for many things to many people too numerous to name here, but it would be falling short of both justice and courtesy were I to omit expressing my debt to many colleagues, past and present, including Dr. Tryphena Humphrey, Dr. Ira D. Hogg, and the staff of the Elizabeth Steel Magee Hospital. The work more specifically presented in the second and part of the third chapters owes much of its financial support to grants from the Penrose Fund of the American Philosophical Society, the Carnegie Foundation of New York, the University of Pittsburgh, the Sarah Mellon Scaife Foundation of Pittsburgh, and the late George Tallman Ladd, also of Pittsburgh.

It is a pleasure to express my indebtedness for many courtesies to Dr. and Mrs. Paul G. Roofe, and to the staff and graduate students in the Department of Anatomy at Kansas. I also wish to thank Mr. Ivan Hird, whose ability as a projectionist made the illustrations for the lectures flow smoothly and accurately.

Contents

Illustrations

The Prenatal Origin of Behavior

Chapter 1

Fetal Activity in Infrahuman Vertebrates

BEHAVIOR IS A fundamental characteristic of all animals, whether adult or developing, unicellular or multicellular. In essence, behavior is the sum total of the adjustments made by the organism to changes in its internal or external environment. The activities of the mechanisms involved in restoring the dynamic balance of the organism as a consequence of the environmental changes give rise to bodily activity, which is the externally visible or overt expression of the functional capacity of the whole organism. In all but the simplest organisms, this activity is produced primarily by the neuromuscular system, but this overt behavior is also influenced by the activities of other systems of the body, which constitute the organism's internal, invisible, or covert behavior. The interacting influences of all the various organ systems of the individual are infinitely complex, so that at any given moment the behavior of the whole organism tends to be different in kind and extent from the sum of the activities of its separate parts.

Structure and function are directly and inseparably related in any living organism. This is as true of one which is developing as it is of the adult. In the embryo, therefore, when any organ reaches a level of development and differentiation consonant with function, it begins to function, provided the environment is appropriate. The qualities of embryonic functioning of an organ may not be those exhibited when its development is complete. Furthermore, all organs do not reach a functional state in their development at the same time. Therefore, the behavior of an organism attains the adult form characteristic of each species only as it approaches maturity.

An embryo develops morphologically in an orderly, sequential manner characteristic of the species. Thus, given an appropriate environment, an organism's behavior also develops in an orderly, sequential manner which, again, is characteristic of its species. However, the morphological development of all vertebrates follows a fundamentally similar sequence. Hence it would be surprising if there were not a similar fundamental sequence of some type in the development of behavior throughout the vertebrate series. A priori, then, one might expect the developmental sequences of behavior in the different vertebrates to possess certain fundamental similarities, but to differ in particulars in different species.

It is this thesis which is to be considered in some detail in the first two chapters. The problem, then, is to survey the origins of behavior, more particularly of the externally visible overt behavior, in developing organisms throughout the vertebrate phylogenetic series. The hope is to establish the points of similarity and of difference between them, if either exist.

The earlier recorded data on embryonic activity consisted largely of casual and uncontrolled observations without experimental attempts to analyze the nature of the movements seen. Although one cannot merely write off earlier observations as worthless, for the observers were both keen and reasonably accurate, nevertheless they were pioneering efforts in a little-understood field and less valuable than those which came later.

It was not until the work of Wilhelm Preyer (1885) that real organization and a scientific approach to the subject appeared. Preyer's interest apparently was stimulated by observations of his own child (1882). However that may be, he gathered together the work of his predecessors in the field and added materially to the then existing state of knowledge by his own wide and exact observations. His work will be noted in the pages which follow.

Important as the work of Preyer was, and there can be no dispute on that point, it was George Ellett Coghill who first placed a firm foundation under the study of embryonic activity. Coghill's work was published in an extraordinary series of 65 papers and one book, from 1898 to the time of his death in 1941. Two of his unpublished manuscripts were posthumously edited by C. Judson Herrick[1] and published. This series of studies laid a solid foundation for the correlation of the development of behavior with the associated changes in the nervous system for the salamander, *Amblystoma*. Coghill's work not only pointed the way for similar studies on other forms, but also stimulated many of his students and some of his associates to continue such investigations.

* * * * * *

One of the first muscular activities exhibited in the vertebrate embryo is the heart beat. The early activity of the heart in vertebrates has been demonstrated to be myogenic in nature in many forms, that is to say, the rhythmic contractility of its musculature is a property inherent in the cardiac muscle cells themselves. Only later in embryonic development do nerves, not yet developed when the cardiac beat begins, control the activity of the heart. The beating of the heart is not ordinarily considered a component of developing behavior. Certainly the heart beat is not a part of the overt behavior of the organism, but an excellent case can be made for its inclusion among the elements of the internal, or covert, behavior of each animal form. It is mentioned here, not to press the latter point, but because similar myogenic movements occur in the trunk musculature of certain forms shortly to be considered in a necessarily rather superficial review of the development of behavior in the infrahuman vertebrate phylogenetic series.

There are three types of movement exhibited by muscles—myogenic, neurogenic, and reflexogenic. As already noted, myogenic activity originates within the muscle tissue itself, without benefit of a nervous or other impulse. Actually the term "myogenic" is used to denote two quite different types of muscle movement. One of these is exhibited spontaneously and, usually, rhythmically. The myogenic heart beat and the rhythmic activities of the axial musculature of fishes are examples. Such myogenic activity is an inherent property of the musculature. The term is also sometimes used, unfortunately and probably inaccurately, to denote muscle movements in response to electrical or mechanical stimulation. In such cases there is a stimulus to the muscle, so that its activity does not have its genesis within the muscle cells as an inherent characteristic of the tissue. When used in that sense in this contribution, the word will be enclosed in quotation marks.

The motor neuron, particularly in embryos, may discharge impulses into muscle tissue, either spontaneously or under the influence of stimuli from outside itself. Such action of motor neurons in activating muscle is termed neurogenic. Again, the term is used for both the inherent spontaneous type of motor discharge and that originating from stimuli to the motor nerve.

In reflexogenic activity, a complete reflex arc—receptor (sensory) neuron, usually one or more intercalated neurons, and an effector (motor) neuron—is involved. Motor neurons appear to establish functional connection with their muscle, ontogenetically, before their sensory or intermediate connections are established. Thus neurogenic action ordinarily ceases when the reflex arc is completed, but it will become evident that in some forms an extension of true spontaneous neurogenic activity may overlap the establishment of reflexogenic activity.

Fishes

Both of the principal investigators of activity in very early selachian embryos, Stewart Paton (1907, 1911) and P. Wintrebert (1920), have given excellent descriptions of the rhythmic contractility of the axial musculature exhibited in these forms. Wintrebert's contribution, perhaps because it succeeded a considerable period of study of the earliest activity in amphibian embryos, offers somewhat more detail and a more complete picture of activity sequences. He has described the side-to-side spontaneous activity of the trunk of one of the cat sharks (*Scylliorhinus canicula*) as first appearing near the end of Stage G, as described by Balfour (1874, 1878). At this stage (G), only one branchial pouch is present. The activity begins as a property of the myotomic tissue, that is to say as a true myogenic phenomenon, of those myotomes capable of muscular contraction. The "aneural" (true myogenic) character of these movements was proved when Wintrebert removed the spinal cord without interrupting the activity. The first movement to appear is often a unilateral flexion of the trunk, moving the head toward either right or left, and a return to the midline. Soon the movement becomes bilateral, first to one side, then to the other, usually as two bilateral swings of the head, each followed by a pause. Because the attachment of the embryo to the yolk sac offers resistance to rotation, the trunk passively returns to its original position during the pause.

The first contractions appear in the more cephalically located myotomes, those first formed in development. Gradually, myotomes behind these begin to participate in the myogenic activity. Without entering into all the details furnished by Wintrebert, one may summarize the characteristics of the side-to-side myotomic contractions as follows: 1) each myotomic movement consists of a lateral flexion of the head and its return to posture, followed by a pause, then, in embryos in which a rhythm has been established, a flexion to the opposite side, and its passive relaxation and pause; 2) the older the embryo, the greater is the number of side-to-side flexions; 3) temperature plays an important role, as the flexions succeed one another more rapidly at the optimum temperature of 15° C. than at higher or lower temperatures, and the time required for a flexion, as well as the duration of the pause, also varies in like manner; and 4) optimum conditions include, not only a temperature of 15° C., but good aeration of the egg-case, proper composition of the sea water in which it is retained, and the absence of disturbing factors.

It is interesting to note that the heart beat in *Scylliorhinus* does not begin until late in Balfour stage I, at which time the myotomes begin to exhibit neurogenic activity, again spreading caudally from those more cephalically located. Still later, reflexogenic activity supervenes.

Paton's (1907, 1911) factual results are, in the main, the same as those of Wintrebert. However, he regarded his results as evidence of the functioning of intercellular protoplasmic bridges capable of transmitting nerve impulses. Hence, he viewed the movements as neurogenic in nature. Hensen (1903) had earlier promulgated the idea that such protoplasmic bridges existed and were, in fact, capable of carrying impulses of a nervous type. Held (1909) had modified the Hensen theory by what he believed to be a demonstration of the formation of neurofibrils in these bridges, which thus became true nerves, a position also held by Graham Kerr (1912). The work of His (1887), Cajal (1906), Harrison (1910), and others has quite definitely proved the nerve fiber to be a protoplasmic outgrowth of the perikaryon of the neuron and not a transformation *in loco* of protoplasmic bridges between body cells. We may safely assume, then, that Paton's findings go to strengthen the interpretation of these early spontaneous movements as being myogenic in character.

Among very young teleosts, somewhat similar spontaneous movements have been observed by Tracy (1925, 1926) in the toadfish (*Opsanus tau*), the cunner (*Tautogolabrus adspersus*), and in several other forms; by Coghill (1933*b*) in the killifish (*Fundulus*) and in the toadfish (unpublished); and by Sawyer (1944) in *Fundulus*. Tracy was at first of the opinion that these bilateral rhythmic axial movements were neurogenic in nature, because he believed that he could demonstrate in *Opsanus* early motor paths in the medulla and cord, "but with the afferent system largely undifferentiated during the earliest stages of motor activity" (1926, pp. 352-53). He thought that these motor nerves might possibly be stimulated to activity by variations in the CO_2 concentration in the embryos (endogenous stimulation), as had White (1915) in her studies on trout embryos. However, as a result of further work, as yet unpublished, he became convinced that they were myogenic in character.

Motility of the trunk first appears in toadfish embryos with 19 to 22 somites in the most cephalic four or five pairs, and the number involved gradually increases caudally. Unlike the side-to-side rhythmic flexions of *Scylliorhinus* described by Wintrebert (1920), the flexions of *Opsanus* are not rhythmic, though they may be grouped, and produce a somewhat coiled state of the body. When these coils are performed alternately from side to side, Tracy termed the responses "flutters" because of their irregular, nonrhythmic nature.

This early myogenic activity persists through hatching, to be followed by a similar cephalocaudally progressing wave of reflexogenous activity. Whether a period of true neurogenic movements exists between the myogenic and reflexogenous periods is as yet uncertain. Tracy believes this sequence is also true of cunner and *Fundulus* embryos.

Tracy's use of "endogenous" as synonymous with "spontaneous" is unfortunate, but the present writer—and many others—have made the same error before the nature of true myogenic or neurogenic movements was as well understood as it is today. Nevertheless, Tracy's 1926 paper performed a major service in once more calling attention to the work of many observers of the effects of CO_2 in appropriate quantities serving to facilitate, though not to originate, activities of the nervous system, a matter to which reference will be made in the third chapter.

Barron (1941) has pointed out that there is no evidence that CO_2 can stimulate a peripheral nerve in such a manner as to initiate neurogenic action. However, if Wintrebert (1920) is correct in his finding that the establishment of a motor nerve connection with a myotome causes its spontaneous contractions to cease, such contractions should be restored, if they are truly myogenic, by the suppressing effect of CO_2 on the nerve.

Coghill's work on the earliest activities of *Opsanus* and *Fundulus* gave support to Tracy's change in viewpoint (see Herrick, 1949, pp. 96-97). Coghill (1933*b*; and see Herrick, 1949, pp. 264-69) divided the early activity of *Fundulus* into five phases, beginning (phase A) with the first localized myogenic contractions of myotomes which became progressively active spontaneously in a general cephalocaudal direction. The wave of myogenic activity, as it spread caudalward in phase B, was shortly replaced (phase C) at the cephalic end of the body by another wave, this one of responses to external stimulation, the initial sensitivity becoming manifest in the area anterior to the eye. In phase D, only the tip of the tail and the pectoral fin still show localized spontaneous activity, which disappears in the last phase (E). Almost identical results were secured by Coghill in *Opsanus*. In both forms, the second or neurogenic wave replaced the myogenic in a caudal direction until, as Coghill expressed it in a letter to Tracy (Herrick, 1949, p. 97), "The neurogenic system chases the myogenic system off the end of the tail, the last of it appearing in the movements of the caudal fin and at the same stage of development in the pectoral fin also." Thus Coghill agreed with Tracy's suggestion that the earliest movements throughout the somatic system were myogenic.

Reflexogenic activity follows the neurogenic in the behavioral sequence, but details are not available, since Coghill's results were never published. Regarding this type of activity, Coghill wrote me in July, 1933, as follows: "I have found that the toadfish, in regard to the individuation of limb reflexes out of a total pattern, fits absolutely with *Amblystoma*, only the period is much longer between the total pattern fin action and fin reflex than in *Amblystoma*."

In his experiments on early *Fundulus* embryos, Coghill used curare, which blocks the motor end-plates of adult organisms. He found that the rhythmic spontaneous movements continued unaffected, and accepted this as clear-cut evidence of their myogenic nature. Barron (1941) criticized, by implication, the curare experiments of Coghill in discussing those of Angulo (1933). Barron's point, with regard to the curare experiments with embryos, was to the effect that the action of curare on immature muscle had never been demonstrated. Its effect might be the same on immature as on adult muscle, but, until proof of this had been offered, any conclusion based on its use that the spontaneous movements of embryos are myogenic was subject to a Scottish verdict of "not proven." However, recent work by Brinley (1951) indicates that curare, in the strengths used by Angulo, Coghill, and Tracy, does act on fish embryonic muscle as it does on that of adults.

On the positive side of the ledger stands the work of Sawyer (1944), whose studies in correlating the type of activity with the cholinesterase (ChE.) content of the embryo, localized chiefly in future muscle and nerve, afford strong evidence that the early spontaneous movements in *Fundulus* are probably myogenic in nature. Sawyer states (1943a) that "cholinesterase content is a biochemical criterion of a phenomenon for which there is no anatomical criterion, i.e., the attainment of functional capacity in the neuromuscular apparatus" (p. 27). He has pointed out that "spontaneous somatic movements begin when there is practically no esterase present and eserine, a ChE. inhibitor, does not affect the movements. They are therefore interpreted as myogenic . . ." (1944, p. 82). This opinion is reinforced by Sawyer's finding that eserine does affect movement when the ChE. levels have risen materially, an occurrence which corresponds with the time true reflexogenic activity is exhibited.

The development of behavior in fishes presents some puzzling problems as yet incompletely resolved. To solve them will require additional studies. Here, especially, there is need for establishing distinctions between myogenic, neurogenic, and reflexogenic activity. At the moment, such distinction is by no means free from ambiguity.

Although the fishes occupy a lowly place in the phylogenetic series, it must not be assumed that they are all necessarily primitive forms. Indeed, many are highly specialized, sometimes along peculiar lines which may well produce unusual developmental behavorial conditions, apparent aberrant types in the theoretical fundamentally similar sequence which we are examining. Also, there is insufficient evidence on reflex behavior. Nevertheless, there is much in the still incomplete knowledge of the development of behavior in the fishes that sustains the idea of such a fundamental sequence, probably at least as much as opposes the idea, even at this time.

Amphibia

In the amphibians, at least in *Amblystoma*, we stand on very sure ground. The work of Coghill (1909-1940) not only laid the most solid foundation for behavioral development existing today in any vertebrate group, but also served to stimulate the majority of subsequent studies on the development of behavior in all vertebrate forms. Consequently, it is essential that we examine his contributions in some detail.

Coghill's studies on *Amblystoma* disclosed several clearly recognizable stages in the development of its activity following two others during which the embryo was inactive. In the first of these two inactive stages, termed the premotile stage, the embryonic myotomic tissue was incapable of contraction. In the second, the nonmotile stage, the myotomes were capable of contraction, but only on direct mechanical or electrical stimulation. Such movements were considered "myogenic," in that they did not originate in the nervous tissue, but they were not spontaneous (see p. 6).

The first of the active stages of *Amblystoma*, termed by Coghill the early flexure stage, represents the first of the neuromuscular responses to external (exteroceptive) stimulation. However, as shown by Preyer (1885) and by Coghill, these movements also appear spontaneously. The first area of embryonic ectoderm to become sensitive to stimulation lies in the neck region over and anterior to the site of later gill formation. As the ectoderm of all young embryos is extremely thin, the method of stimulation is of great importance, because too stiff a stimulator (esthesiometer) may directly stimulate the underlying muscle tissue either by pressure or by actual penetration. Coghill used a human hair which he stroked lightly over the sensitive area. It can thus be seen that the stiffness of the stimulator must be correlated with the thickness of the epidermis of the embryo stimulated.

When the sensitive area of ectoderm in an *Amblystoma* embryo in the early flexure stage is properly stimulated with a human hair the response is characteristic and stereotyped. "Stereotyped" is intended to convey the concept that each response is, within the general limits of variation of biological processes, practically identical with every other, so that they are patterned and constant within that pattern. The greatest variation found by Coghill consisted in occasional flexions toward the side stimulated, although the almost constant finding was a contralateral flexion.

The early flexure response to stimulation within the sensitive area consists of a flexion in the neck region, so that the head almost forms a right angle with the long axis of the body (fig. 1) and in the vast majority of cases does this toward the side opposite that stimulated. When this response first appears, the flexure at the neck is somewhat less than a right angle and the contracting myotomes are few in number. As development proceeds, more myotomes, located caudally from those initially contracting, become functional and the flexure becomes more marked.

It must be borne in mind that the development of activity is always a continuous process and that any division into phases or stages is entirely artificial. The whole process is a smoothly progressive affair and not a series of isolated posturings. Consequently, the transition from the early flexure to the coil, Coghill's second stage, is characterized by the spread caudally of the flexion, as more and more

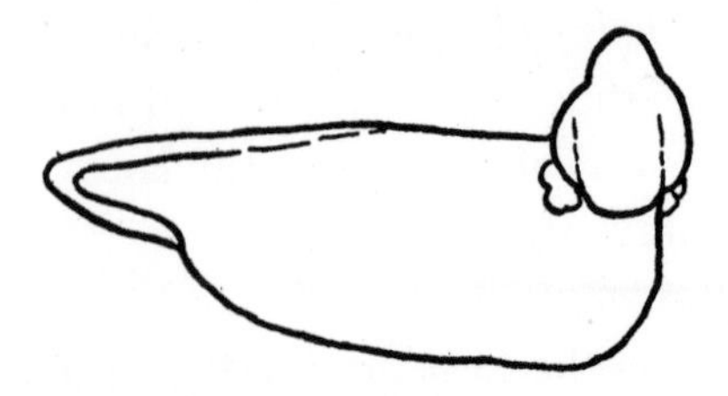

Fig. 1. Early flexure stage of *Amblystoma*. Outline drawn by projection of the original Swenson-Coghill film. (By permission of the Wistar Institute of Anatomy and Biology.)

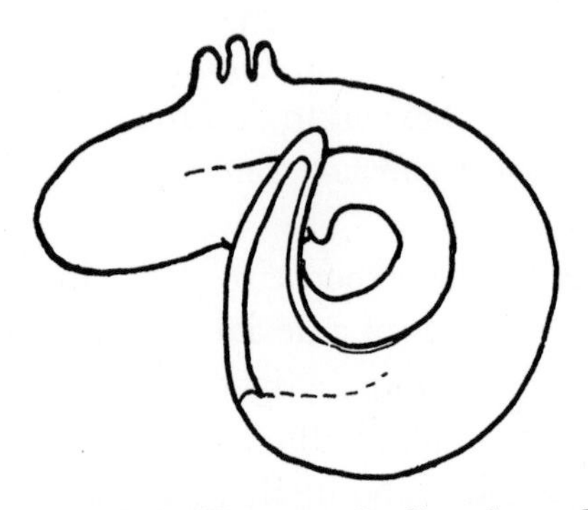

Fig. 2. Coil stage of *Amblystoma*. Outline drawn by projection from the original Swenson-Coghill film. (By permission of the Wistar Institute of Anatomy and Biology.)

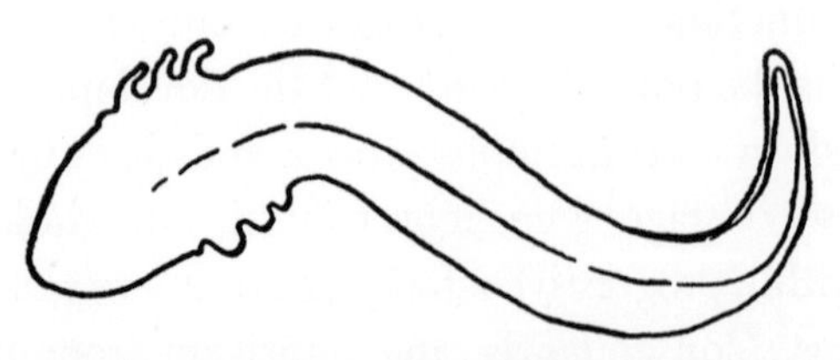

Fig. 3. S-response of *Amblystoma*. Outline drawn by projection from the original Swenson-Coghill film. (By permission of the Wistar Institute of Anatomy and Biology.)

myotomes become functional, until the entire trunk is coiled to the contralateral side, with the tail overlapping the head (fig. 2). The coil results from a briefly maintained contraction of the myotomes of the side opposite to that stimulated.

For the third stage, the S-reaction (fig. 3), new neural mechanisms, in the form of collaterals, are thrown into action. Although the appearance of the S-response is relatively sudden, the collaterals which make it possible have been developing toward a functional stage for some time. Herrick and Coghill (1915) and Coghill (1916, 1924a, 1929) worked out the neural mechanisms for the various stages. Coghill's generalized diagram (1924a, fig. 43) is here reproduced in a slightly modified form (fig. 4). It will be noted that the afferent mechanism begins with general sensory components carried in the fifth, seventh, and tenth cranial nerves. Although the last two nerves named contribute little in the early stages, the trigeminal fibers enter the descending tract of that nerve, as will those from the facial and vagus later. The trigeminal general sensory fibers have early grown caudally to synapse with tract neurons of the spinal cord. This is in agreement with Coghill's (1902) findings in adult *Amblystoma*. Stimuli perceived in front of the ear are transmitted as impulses over these general cutaneous fibers. Behind the ear, sensations are picked up by the cutaneous elements of the Rohon-Beard cells, and their impulses enter the ascending sensory path as it develops. All impulses are transmitted across to the contralateral side of the cord by the floor plate cells, shown in the middle of the diagram, thus causing contralateral responses.

Essentially, the S-reaction is an outgrowth of the coil

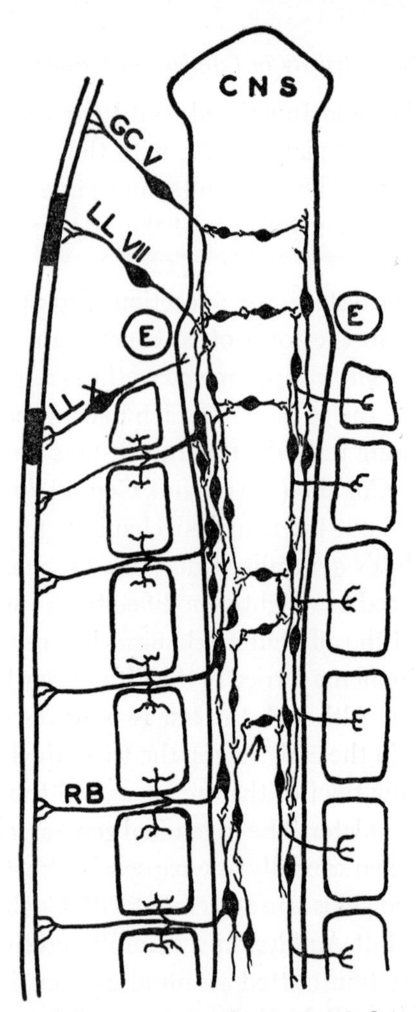

FIG. 4. Diagram of the nervous mechanism underlying the early behavior pattern of *Amblystoma*. (After Coghill, 1924a, fig. 43.)

The afferent paths are given on the left side of the figure, connected by six floor-plate commissural cells (center) to the motor pathway shown on the right side. Description is in the text, page 17. Abbreviations used: *CNS*, outline of the central nervous system; *E*, ear; *GC* V, general cutaneous component of the fifth (trigeminal) nerve which enters the descending tract of that nerve; *LL VII* and *LL X*, lateral line branches of the seventh (facial) and tenth (vagus) nerves, which contain general cutaneous components, later to course with those of the trigeminal in the latter's descending tract; *RB*, Rohon-Beard cells, mediating both cutaneous and muscle sense.

response, but with a difference. As the coil develops by the rapid caudalward progression of the motor component of the reflex, a transfer of the wave from the contralateral to the ipsilateral side of the trunk occurs in the neck region. Thus, as the now slowed contraction wave passes caudally on one side of the body, a new contraction begins in the cervical area on the other side and progresses caudally in its turn. This throws the trunk into the form of the letter *S* momentarily, but as each contraction wave passes off the tail on one side, another starts cephalically on the same side, thus alternating with that of the opposite side (fig. 3). The trunk, then, undergoes a series of sinuous movements in a head-to-tail direction, which, when they become sufficiently rapid and strong, move the embryo forward in the early swimming stage. At this time, no limbs are present.

At this juncture, it seems advisable to return to the mechanisms of the earlier stages, for they represent the basis for Coghill's concept of the "total pattern" response. There has been so much misunderstanding of what he meant by that term that some further consideration should be given to it here.

Coghill found that the sensitive area of the ectoderm was at first strictly localized and that, on the motor side, all of the myotomes which were capable of being excited to contraction by their motor nerves participated in the response. Inasmuch as only those in the cervical region were so prepared for action at first, the early flexure stage resulted, but as more and more neuromuscular mechanism became functional caudally, the early flexure widened into the coil. In other words, there was a total response of all functional neuromuscular apparatus. Coghill termed it a "total pattern" response. The total pattern persists far beyond these early responses, however, and in *Amblystoma* remains dominant throughout the life of the organism.

As has already been noted, these responses in the normal embryo are true reflexes. Weiss (1941*a*, 1941*b*,), however, has demonstrated that amphibian embryos with the dorsal spinal roots cut along both sides of the entire spinal cord may swim in perfect co-ordination. Herrick and Coghill at first (1915) inclined to the opinion that proprioceptive stimuli played an essential role in producing the S-reaction. Later (1926*b*) Coghill recognized that the neural mechanism governing this alternation of contraction waves on the two sides of the body might lie within the motor system entirely, though he believed the proprioceptive field facilitated the duration of the response. It would appear that, under normal conditions and in response to exteroceptive stimuli, the responses are reflexogenic, but that, under abnormal conditions, activities may be actually neurogenic in origin. This appears to be the chief evidence of actual neurogenic activity in the Amphibia. It has not been demonstrated as a separate type, as is the case, apparently, in fishes,[2] unless the early spontaneous activity should prove to be neurogenic, which seems unlikely.

Following the early swimming stage, at about the beginning of which the *Amblystoma* larvae ordinarily hatch, any true staging is difficult. The larvae then begin to develop along multiple lines, one of which is toward feeding and another toward walking. As the limbs develop, they are at first used solely as a part of the trunk muscle system, having no power of independent movement. Indeed, even after specific limb movements appear, locomotion on land continues to involve the trunk, and in swimming the extremities are streamlined alongside the body. As the gills develop, they also move with the trunk before independent movements are possible. Each new structural complex, as it begins to function, is at first co-ordinated with the trunk as a part of the total pattern, only later coming to possess the capacity for independent motion. This secondary acquisition of the capacity for local movements Coghill spoke of as the "individuation of partial patterns from the total pattern."

In Coghill's opinion, the initial movements exhibited are total patterns which expand by shunting into the neural mechanism previously completely integrated additional elements. Integration is thus a primary phenomenon occurring during neural development.

Much more might be said regarding Coghill's work, but neither space nor time permits. It is essential, however, that Coghill's fundamental conclusions be presented in some detail to establish the basic tenets of his concept of the development of behavior. We have already seen that he believed his concept to hold good for the fishes, and it will become evident in subsequent pages that many persons, a goodly number of whom were not his students, have come to the conclusion that it also applies to other forms. Even those who have considered his ideas as having no validity for so-called higher forms, accept them for *Amblystoma*. Certainly no other series of conclusions has been based upon such detailed and adequate evidence.

It now becomes desirable to present briefly other important studies on the development of activity in the Amphibia. Preyer (1885), in his remarkable book already mentioned, presents his observations on the spontaneous movements of frog (*Rana*) embryos within the egg. Little has been said about spontaneous movements in *Amblystoma* so far, but they occur, as noted by Coghill repeatedly (1930*b* and elsewhere). Unlike this phenomenon in the fishes and in the amniotic contractions in birds, spontaneous movements in the Amphibia are not myogenic, but are certainly either neurogenic or reflexogenic. The whole question of spontaneous movements is as yet incompletely resolved. Such movements may be caused by unrecognized stimuli of various types or they may arise, quite independently of stimuli, as an inherent property of nervous substance, as has been pointed out by Weiss (1941*a*, 1941*b*, 1941*c*) and noted earlier. Preyer's work, unfortunately but not unexpectedly, throws little light on this aspect of the problem. Nevertheless, his observations on sequence of activities are quite accurate.

Youngstrom (1938) presented the results of a careful study of the activities of embryos of *Rana, Bufo, Pseudacris,* and *Acris*. He found surprising agreement in the nature (though differences in time consumed in attaining it) of the activity sequence in these anurans, which he details as follows: 1) spontaneous bending of the head, characterized by slow contraction and relaxation, at a time when any form of external stimulation is ineffective in causing a response: 2) deep pressure stimulation, suddenly applied, presumably in the branchial area, caused responses in which the body was bent, often ipsilaterally, into an arc, which he regards as the equivalent of Coghill's coil stage; 3) again with quick deep pressure, the appearance of a double wave of contraction forming a kind of S-reaction, the amount of yolk present in the shorter trunk of anurans probably accounting for the differences in these last two responses from those of *Amblystoma*; and then 4) irregular swimming movements; later, 5) to light touch stimulation, the S and, soon after, swimming movements occurred, the sensitive area being at first over the side of the head, gradually increasing caudalward over the trunk and finally reaching the tail. Youngstrom concludes that "the Coghillian sequence of developing behavior has been found to apply, with only slight variation, to the *Anura*" (1938, p. 372).

Wang and Lu (1940, 1941), working on *Rana* and *Bufo*, also agreed with the general outline of activity as described by Coghill for *Amblystoma*, but more exactly with Youngstrom's work on *Anura*. They describe six successive stages, viz: 1) nonmotile; 2) flexure; 3) S-reaction; 4) "translatory body movements"; corresponding to Youngstrom's "irregular swimming"; 5) controlled swimming; and 6) the appearance and maintenance of the upright position when at rest, as well as in motion, with the definite presence of righting reflexes. In addition to their observations on the sequence of appearance of responses in normal embryos, they transected the central nervous system at various levels, with instructive results. Removal of, or section behind, the forebrain or diencephalon had no effect on the sequence of appearance of activity throughout the embryonic period. Transection at the caudal border of the mesencephalon prevented development of righting reflexes or maintenance of upright posture. Cord section at any level arrested the appearance of swimming. Furthermore, spinal, decerebrate, or mesencephalic tadpoles exhibited spontaneous movements, although adult anurans, so operated upon, do not.

Cholinesterase (ChE.) determinations for *Ambly-*

stoma, *Rana*, and *Bufo* have been made by Youngstrom (1938), and for *Amblystoma* alone by Sawyer (1943*a*, 1943*b*) and by Boell and Shen (1950). Youngstrom found a significant increase in ChE. concentration in all three forms during the period of increasing activity. Sawyer reported that a small amount of ChE. was present in actual or presumptive nerve and muscle tissues even in premotile embryos, that the quantity of ChE. increases in nerve and muscle during the swimming stages and reaches its highest peak at the feeding period, when activity is greatest, gradually falling off in amount to the adult level. Boell and Shen found that ChE. first appears in the spinal cord at about Harrison stage 36,[3] when the embryo is capable of responding to tactile stimulation. Gradually, detectable amounts of ChE. appear, caudocephalically, in the hindbrain (stage 38), midbrain (stage 39), and in the forebrain (stage 42 or later). They believe that the increase in ChE. is correlated with functional differentiation rather than with mere increase in size and that the amount present forms a gradient with the highest concentration in the cord, decreasing steadily in a cephalic direction.

The importance of these observations, even though they do not always agree in details, cannot be overestimated. Cholinesterase depolarizes the nerve fiber after passage of a nervous impulse over it. Its presence in appreciable quantity, therefore, indicates that nerve activity is at least possible.

In summary, it may be said that the Amphibia present a clear-cut case for the total-pattern idea of the development of behavior. This is based largely upon the classic studies of Coghill on *Amblystoma*, but is supported as a principle by all other investigators on amphibian forms. It would appear that there is reasonable agreement, although with expected variations, in the nature of behavioral development in the tailed and tailless forms. Furthermore, Coghill's basic work is accepted by almost all those who have worked in the field.

Reptiles

Very little work has been done on the development of behavior in any reptilian forms other than the turtles. Emmert and Hochstetter (1811) on lizards, Valenciennes (1841) on python, and Preyer (1885) on ring adders appear to have presented the only (and meager) data on other forms. This is an area where a great need for facts exists.

Tuge (1931), working with terrapin embryos, observed spontaneous movements before exteroceptive stimulation was effective. When the embryos are about 6 mm. in length, the first sensitivity to external stimuli appears on the snout. The response is a contralateral flexion of the head and neck. Very soon thereafter the response spreads caudally to involve the trunk, tail, and extremities, but the limbs are not themselves sensitive at this time and do not move independently of the trunk until the embryos are between 7 and 7.5 mm. in length. At this stage the extremities become sensitive to stimulation, and both the fore and hind limbs begin independent movement at the same time.

Coghill (see Herrick, 1949, pp. 100 and 253) had observed the studies by Tuge and confirmed each of his points.

Smith and Daniel (1946) have published a preliminary report of their studies on embryos of the loggerhead turtle, *Caretta caretta*. Their results are of considerable interest. Before the shell is more than a soft, dorsally located swelling, they observed a "mass movement" (total pattern) type of activity at 12 to 14 days, in the form of an abortive kind of C-response, the head flexing to the concave side, both on stimulation and spontaneously. At this time the limbs did not participate, but moved, by 18 to 21 days, with the trunk as part of the total pattern. Specific reactions became evident at 22 days, when the shell was present in sufficient mass to prevent trunk movements. These specific responses occurred first in the eyelids, mouth, and head, as a whole, to be followed at 24 or 25 days by independent limb movements.

Professor Smith has been kind enough to supply additional details on the site of effective stimulation and the nature of the C-response. When first manifested, the most effective site for the reception of stimuli is the integument over the head, with no specific localization, and the base of the flippers comes next. The earliest C-responses have no consistent direction, ipsilateral or contralateral, in relation to the side stimulated, but after five to seven days, when the carapace has developed further, they tend to become ipsilateral. At that time, head extension has replaced lateral flexion, so that the head-trunk movements have become a "dual twisting of the head and body."

Between 26 and 32 days, activities appeared in the following sequence: 1) co-ordinated swimming by limb action, 2) snapping of the jaws, 3) nystagmic head movements when the embryo was rotated, 4) righting movements, and 5) crawling. As these turtles do not hatch until the 45th to 50th day, all of these activities occurred in embryos removed from the egg.

The evidence available on reptiles, and this is actually limited to observations on turtles, indicates that these highly specialized forms present a Coghillian type of sequence modified by the rapid development of the carapace. It is indeed unfortunate that no detailed studies have been made recently on lizard embryos which may prove the least specialized of these interesting animals.

Birds

Bird embryos have intrigued observers greatly over the ages. Among the earliest recorded studies are those of William Harvey (1651), who observed movements on the 6th day of incubation of the chick. Beguelin (1757) was possibly the first to record the peculiar myogenic movements of the amnion, a nerveless membrane which pulsates more or less rhythmically at an early time. Von Baer (1828) and Remak (1854) observed similar movements of the yolk sac of the chick, and Vulpian (1857) demonstrated that they may subsequently be found also in the allantois.

Most of the other early observations are of little moment for our purposes, but it might be mentioned here that Home (1822) recorded the first limb movements, and von Baer (1828) very carefully reported the activities of the 6th to the 16th day, which were confirmed by Remak (1854).

The chick egg, like other bird eggs, affords deceptively easy access to the embryo. The difficulties lie not in exposing the embryo but in maintaining it in a normally living state while under observation for any extended period. These difficulties were recognized by various investigators, and some made efforts to overcome or avoid them. To this end, both Vulpian (1857) and Preyer (1885) observed the developing embryo through the unopened shell by transluminating the egg. It is amazing that they secured so many results by this method, for Vulpian saw both the amniotic and bodily movements of the chick embryo, and Preyer was able to list the sequence of a considerable number of activities, albeit his timing of the eggs was slightly inaccurate according to later observations. His series of recorded activities presents a good continuous pattern of developmental behavior which in many respects suggests a Coghillian type sequence. Clark and Clark (1914), working on lymph heart pulsations, confirmed most of Preyer's observations.

The three important recent contributors to the study of the activities of bird embryos are Kuo (1932 to 1939), Tuge (1934, 1937), and Windle and his co-workers (1934 to 1938). Kuo and Windle *et al.* worked on the chick, Tuge on the pigeon.

Kuo utilized a very ingenious technic to make his continuous observations possible. After carefully chipping away the shell from the large end of the egg where the air space is located, he vaselined the membrane to render it moderately transparent. Strong translumination of the shell made possible not only direct observation of the embryo, but also the taking of motion pictures of unexpected clarity. At the same time, the egg could be incubated in the usual manner. He used several thousand eggs in his studies.

Kuo reported that the chick heart begins to beat at about 36 hours of incubation. As the heart increased in size, its beat caused "vibrations" of the head and body by 66 hours, head lifting at 68 hours, head bending at 70 hours, trunk movements at 84 hours, and head turning at 90 hours. The complications attending analysis of the nature of the movements observed as a result of the general upheaval of the embryo by the heart beat are further increased, from 86 hours on, by the appearance of amniotic contractions. The difficulties of such an analysis are much like attempting to determine whether movements exhibited by a flexible object floating in the ocean during a storm at sea originate within the object itself or are caused by the environment. Kuo believed that the activity of the heart and later of the amnion passively excites these spontaneous activities of the embryo.

In the latter part of the fourth day of incubation, Kuo (1932a) states that reflexogenic activity begins as a spontaneous phenomenon, the movements of the amnion and yolk sac serving as the source of stimulation. These reflexes increase in frequency at first with increase in age. The sequence of appearance of reflex activities is cephalocaudal in direction and their character tends to parallel the earlier non-reflex movements until after the 14th day, when the myogenic activity of amnion and yolk sac, and the spontaneous reflexes excited by it, cease. The reflex activities appear in the following order: 1) head bending, 2) trunk "bending," extension and twisting, 3) head turning, 4) forelimb movements, then responses of 5) hind limbs, 6) tail, 7) beak, 8) toes, 9) eyelids, 10) eyeballs, 11) swallowing, 12) bill clapping, 13) trunk wriggling, and 14) trunk rotation.

Although not too sympathetic to Coghill's views, Kuo himself (1932a) states that the earliest response pattern found by him "agrees with Coghill's ('29) observation." However, Kuo fails to make careful distinctions between the presumably myogenic early movements and later possibly neurogenic or definitely reflexogenic activities. The reflexes, as their development is described by Kuo, do form a Coghillian sequence, but the embryo's movements show a progressive reduction in their frequency and amplitude after the ninth day, at which time response to tactile stimulation first appears. Responses to pressure were, however, observed earlier (5th day) in some embryos.

Kuo (1939) was able to demonstrate the presence of acetylcholine in chick embryos at 60 hours, but no evidence of the presence of cholinesterase has been provided. Kuo states that he could determine no evidence that the presence of acetylcholine had any effect upon the development of reflexes.

Preyer believed that the chick embryo spontaneously exhibited a kind of C-shaped trunk flexion at the time amniotic movements began, but Kuo fails to note any such action. The latter recorded a series of spontaneous movements as appearing in the following order: active limb movements at 90 hours, when the head turned, also spontaneously; tail movements at 92 hours; neck flexion at 96 hours; independent, active, but irregular movements of head, trunk, tail, and limbs at 115 hours; opening and closing of the bill at 7 days; and swallowing a day later.

The embryos exhibited responses to electrical stimuli by 90 to 100 hours but did not exhibit responses to deep pressure until about 144 hours. Local limb reflexes were elicited at 155 hours, and respiratory movements began at 15 to 18 days.

Tuge (1934, 1937) worked out the sequence of activity in the carrier pigeon. At 85 hours, the embryos begin to exhibit generalized wave-like spontaneous movements, believed to be myogenic in type because curare does not abolish them. These persist until the sixth day. At 95 hours, there are superimposed upon these spontaneous movements others which are eliminated by curare. These movements, spontaneous flexions of the neck and head, may be unilateral or, in a few cases, bilateral and are considered by Tuge to be neurogenic in nature. These spontaneous flexions expand caudally to include the trunk (101 hours), the rump (115 hours), the tail (120 hours), and the extremities with the trunk (125 hours) and, finally, independent tail and limb movements (133 hours). This type of activity ceases between 135 and 144 hours.

In the meantime, responses to stimulation of "snout" or upper neck with a human hair begin at 123 hours in the form of flexions of the head, neck, and trunk. The reflexogenous zone of the skin spreads in the following sequence: "snout," neck, trunk, back, and hip by 133 hours. Similarly, the reaction pattern expands caudally to hip with trunk (125 hours), tail with trunk (130 hours), and extremities (depending on which is stimulated) with the trunk (133 hours). Independent tail reflexes were observed at 145 hours and of the extremities at 150 hours. Thus, Tuge's results agree with the concept of a true Coghillian sequence.

Another, but less extensive, series of observations on bird embryos are those of Windle with his collaborators (1934 to 1938), carried out on the chick. These investigators have presented analyses of the spontaneous motility, and that in response to mechanical (tapping the embryo or "flipping" the limb with a blunt fiber needle) and electrical (faradic) stimuli.

The sequence of spontaneous activity is listed as given below by Orr and Windle (1934). The first time given represents the initial appearance of the particular type of activity, the second that at which a majority of embryos exhibit it. The sequence is: 1) ventroflexion of the trunk, 4½ to 5½ days; 2) lateral flexion of the trunk, 5½ to 6 days; 3) "swimming" type of activity, 5½ to 6½ days; 4) movement of the tail with the trunk, 5½ to 8 days; 5) movement of the extremities with the trunk, 7 to 8 days; 6) independent movement of the extremities, 7½ to 9 days; and 7) independent movements of the tail, 8 days in some. It will be noted that the time of occurrence of these activities is later than that given by Kuo and by Tuge, though it is sometimes difficult to match performance in the several studies. This is, perhaps, only a semantic difficulty.

In response to mechanical stimulation of the types used, generalized responses to trunk stimulation occurred at 6 to 9 days; local wing reflexes to wing stimulation at 6 to 7½ days; generalized "writhing" of the trunk to wing stimulation at 6½ to 9 days; local leg reflexes to leg stimulation at 7 to 8 days; generalized "writhing" of the trunk to leg stimulation at 7½ days in some; and either local or generalized response to "snout" stimulation at 7 to 9 days. Here again, quite aside from the adequacy or inadequacy of the stimulation used for analysis of the different types of activity elicitable, the terms used to describe the responses have a confusing, rather than a clarifying, effect. In response to faradic current stimulation, local muscular contractions were secured at 6 to 6½ days. That they were not found earlier is puzzling, since ventral and lateral flexions of the trunk occurred by 5 days.

Windle and Orr (1934) believe that when these trunk flexions occurred spontaneously at about 5 days, the sensory elements of the possible reflex arc were only "very feebly developed," and that there were no association neuronal connections present. Some 12 hours later, when spontaneous bilateral trunk flexions were observed, the ventral longitudinal pathway of the cord was connected with the motor paths by collaterals into the mantle layer. They report that at 6 days, when their type of "mechanical stimulation" first became effective in the form of unilateral wing reflexes, collaterals from the dorsal funiculus entered the alar plate mantle layer, and they believe that this is the channel of reflex action at this time. Although the spinal accessory nerve (XI) is believed to function in the earlier reflexes, afferent fibers in the dorsal roots are presumed to take over behind the second cervical level.

The birds constitute a very difficult group in which to study the sequence of activity in development. This is true for several reasons, most notable of which is the constant motion imparted to the entire embryo by the beating of the relatively large heart and by the contractions of the amnion and allantois. Presumably, except for the definitely myogenic character of the amniotic contractions, all of the early spontaneous body activities are at least neurogenic, but proof is still lacking. Whether or not the sequence of activity is Coghillian in nature is strongly contested by the several investigators. What is needed here is further study unbiased by preconceived ideas as to what the results should demonstrate. Such studies can be made. The difficulties to be overcome are not as formidable as those encountered in the work on mammalian embryos.

Infrahuman Mammals

Historically, except for the work of Preyer (1885) and Lane (1917), systematic studies on the developmental sequence of activity in the infrahuman mammals began while Coghill's investigations on *Amblystoma* were still in progress. The work of Swenson and Angulo, actually the first of the more recent mammalian behavioral studies, were carried out at Kansas under Coghill's direction. Only Tracy's studies on the fishes were contemporaneous.

Preyer (1885) published the results of a rather extensive series of observations on the embryonic development of activity in the guinea pig. Although his observations were conducted with care and a keen eye, he overlooked the rapid cooling of the embryo or fetus. This is a most important consideration which may be overcome quite readily and which causes a rapid rise in the threshold to stimulation and earlier failure of the neuromuscular response of the organism being observed. The other factor was the hypoxic condition permitted to supervene. In some forms, hypoxia may be overcome only with great difficulty and, per se, is far less important than cooling. However, failure to take these factors into consideration tends to detract from the significance of the results secured.

The work of several other investigators should be mentioned here, although, for one reason or another, their work is of less importance for the purposes of this review. Lane (1917) studied the development of function, in relation to structure, of the special senses of the albino rat. Avery's (1928) studies on guinea-pig fetuses were limited to older ages, as was the work of Tilney and Kubie (1931) and of Tilney (1933) on the interrelation of brain structure and level of activity exhibited in cat and rat embryos. Originally projected to include a study of embryos of the opossum, the guinea pig, and man as well, the investigations were incomplete because of the death of the senior investigator.

The initial modern work on the Mammalia was instituted by Coghill in the Department of Anatomy at Kansas as a part of his program of covering most of the vertebrate classes, and at about the time Tracy began his studies on *Opsanus*. The plan was for two of his graduate students to attack the problem in rat embryos, one, Swenson, to study the physiological responses, the other, Angulo, to do the morphological part of the investigation.

In his University of Kansas Ph.D. thesis (1926),[4] unfortunately never published, Swenson detailed a series of six successive response types exhibited by the rat embryo between the initiation of reflex activity on the 16th day and the 18th day after insemination. This series began with a contralateral flexion of the neck, trunk, and rump at 378 hours, passed through a stage of lateral flexions of this type alternating from side to side, followed in turn by forelimb flexion and extension, hind limb abduction and adduction, dorso-ventral extension-flexion movements, first apparent in the head and then extending to the trunk, and rump rotation with tail and thigh extension, the last on the 18th day. In a report to the American Association of Anatomists in 1928, Swenson somewhat modified his succession of trunk movements into a series as follows: 1) unilateral trunk flexions, 2) head extension, 3) ventral rump flexion, 4) head rotation, and 5) rump rotation.

It must be borne in mind that these observations were of a pioneering nature. Until experience has been gained by a long series of observations, it is difficult to analyze what has been seen. Furthermore Swenson, in addition to the usual method of stroking the embryo with a hair, adopted two types of stimulation which complicate interpretation of the reactions. One of these was to clamp the umbilical cord. This procedure causes frantic bodily movements in young subprimate fetuses, though in human embryos and fetuses no such response follows clamping of the umbilical cord. The other was the use of stiff stimulators to "flip" a limb. By forcibly extending a limb and then allowing it to return to position with a sudden jerk, very early limb movements secondary to the "flip" may be secured. Although such movements can be elicited at about the time activity in response to true exteroceptive stimuli occurs, Swenson believed them proprioceptive in nature. Coghill, however, was of the opinion that they were the result of direct muscle stimulation. Actually, either explanation may be valid, in the absence of morphological evidence. To set in motion stretch reflexes, usually considered to be bineuronal, requires far less muscle elongation than that provided by the limb-flip.

In 1929, Swenson, who had left the Wistar Institute for the Department of Anatomy at Pennsylvania, adopted a "simple movement" plus "simple movement" idea with the statement, "Each simple movement makes its first appearance in a definite order with relation to the other simple movements." He then believed that the order of appearance of movements had to do with three successive categories, namely: progression, respiration, and ingestion of food. Unfortunately, this seems a marked oversimplification not borne out by the work of others.

After Swenson left the Wistar Institute, Angulo took over the survey of physiological stages (1932-1951). His studies on the morphological aspects of the nervous system were published from 1927 to 1932. In his studies on the development of motility in the rat, Angulo (1932*b*) established four major phases: 1) the nonmotile, 2) the "myogenic," 3) the neurogenic, and 4) the reflex. The non-motile phase ends at about 360 hours (15th day), to be followed by the "myogenic." The "myogenic" responses are not spontaneous, but are manifested on mechanical or electrical stimulation of the muscle tissue. The "myogenic" phase is very brief, lasting in general not more than 10 hours and followed by another, even briefer period of neurogenic activity.

Between the 378th and 380th hour, reflex activity appears in response to stroking the snout region with a light hair. The first response is a contralateral flexion of the trunk, especially in the neck and upper trunk region. In all, Angulo was able to establish a series of 30 responses (tables 1 and 2). Examination of these responses demonstrates that they form a well-integrated Coghillian sequence, even though in some details it differs from that exhibited by other mammalian forms, as we shall see. This is, however, to be expected and it is impossible to overemphasize the fact that each species of vertebrate has its own variations in sequence, insofar as details are concerned.

Pankratz (1931), in the course of a study on the development of the adrenal gland in the rabbit, reported in a preliminary contribution six steps in the development of its overt behavior. These were: 1) lateral flexion of the neck and upper trunk (15 to 16 days), 2) ventroflexion of the neck and upper trunk with some movement of the forelimbs as part of the trunk response (17 days), and by the 20th day, 3) opening and closing of the mouth, 4) independent movements of the forelimbs, 5) hind limb flexion, and 6) lateral flexion of the entire trunk. So far as information is given, we have here a reasonable Coghillian

TABLE 1

Index to nature of each response secured by A. W. Angulo, 1932*b*, listed in table 2.

(By permission of the author and of the Wistar Institute of Anatomy and Biology.)

0. non-motile
1, lateral flexion of the trunk
2, lateral flexion of the trunk with movement of the fore limbs
3, lateral flexion of the rump
4, extension of the head
5, extension of the head with opening of the mouth
6, extension of the head with opening of the mouth and protrusion of the tongue
7, lateral flexion of the rump with movement of the hind limbs
8, ventroflexion of the trunk and rump
9, independent movement of the fore limbs
10, maintained contractions
11, contraction of the abdominal muscles
12, extension of the rump
13, flexion at the elbow and wrist associated with trunk movements
14, attempt to assume "the optimum physiological posture"
15, rotation of the trunk and rump
16, independent movement of the hind limbs
17, extension of the head and rump with kicking of the hind limbs
18, independent opening of the mouth
19, independent extension of the hands
20, independent flexion of the hands
21, specific reflexes
22, movement of the tail
23, flexion at the ankle
24, wrinkling of the skin
25, flexion of the hip
26, movement of the toes
27, independent movement of the feet
28, independent movement of the tongue
29, wrinkling of the snout
30, independent active closing of the mouth

sequence, though one differing in details from that described by Angulo in the rat.

Coronios (1933), working on cat embryos, observed still other variations in the order of development of activity (table 3). His method of stimulation, a light brush, is good but allows less information concerning exact localization than does a light hair. The sequence of appearance of reflex activity presented by Coronios actually lends considerable support to the Coghillian total pattern idea, although neither Coronios nor Carmichael, under whose direction the work was done, was sympathetic to the total pattern concept. One of the difficulties in the interpretation of these results is again semantic. "Retraction" of a limb can be its extension, abduction, or adduction. Apparently only training in human anatomy, with its exact terminology of the nature of different movements, affords the desirable background for avoiding this difficulty.

Carmichael (1934) made an extensive study of the guinea pig embryo from 27 to 67 postcopulation days for areas sensitive to various types of stimulation. He used punctiform stimulation and stroke with a "pliable" hair, pressure with a "strong" bristle or blunt probe, pricking

TABLE 2

Percentage of responses at indicated ages in the rat embryo and fetus, from Angulo, 1932*b*. (By permission of the Wistar Institute of Anatomy and Biology.)

REACTIONS	14 DAYS	15 DAYS	16 DAYS	17 DAYS	18 DAYS	19 DAYS	20 DAYS	21 DAYS
0	100	68	29					
1		32	71	71	36	7		
2			59	92	66	52	52	100
3			43	54	35	13		
4			7	81	96	89	72	100
5			35	74	58	27		
6			10	22	43	26		
7			5	49	53	67		
8			8	54	38	31	28	45
9			1?	42	42	26	20	80
10			2?	8	77	89	72	45
11				54	38	31	28	45
12				30	47	90	75	100
13				18				
14				9	23	24	65	45
15				21	34	18		
16				10	16	20	27	100
17				5	53	89	70	100
18					30	20	22	45
19					52	79	96	100
20					48	78	96	100
21					30	79	96	100
22					11	16		40
23					11			
24					4	2		
25					3	2		
26								
27						4	65	65
28					3?		52	65
29						51	83	60
30						13	42	100

TABLE 3

Table of responses in the cat fetus, from Coronios, 1933. (By permission of The Journal Press.)

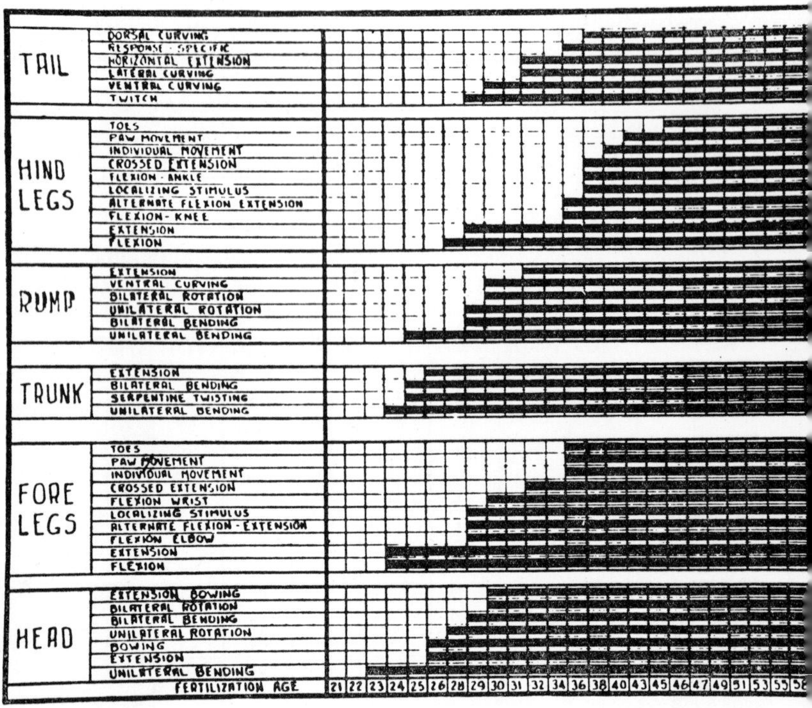

TAIL	DORSAL CURVING
	RESPONSE - SPECIFIC
	HORIZONTAL EXTENSION
	LATERAL CURVING
	VENTRAL CURVING
	TWITCH
HIND LEGS	TOES
	PAW MOVEMENT
	INDIVIDUAL MOVEMENT
	CROSSED EXTENSION
	FLEXION - ANKLE
	LOCALIZING STIMULUS
	ALTERNATE FLEXION EXTENSION
	FLEXION - KNEE
	EXTENSION
	FLEXION
RUMP	EXTENSION
	VENTRAL CURVING
	BILATERAL ROTATION
	UNILATERAL ROTATION
	BILATERAL BENDING
	UNILATERAL BENDING
TRUNK	EXTENSION
	BILATERAL BENDING
	SERPENTINE TWISTING
	UNILATERAL BENDING
FORE LEGS	TOES
	PAW MOVEMENT
	INDIVIDUAL MOVEMENT
	CROSSED EXTENSION
	FLEXION WRIST
	LOCALIZING STIMULUS
	ALTERNATE FLEXION - EXTENSION
	FLEXION ELBOW
	EXTENSION
	FLEXION
HEAD	EXTENSION BOWING
	BILATERAL ROTATION
	BILATERAL BENDING
	UNILATERAL ROTATION
	BOWING
	EXTENSION
	UNILATERAL BENDING
	FERTILIZATION AGE: 21, 22, 23, 24, 25, 26, 28, 29, 30, 31, 32, 34, 36, 38, 40, 43, 45, 46, 47, 49, 51, 53, 55, 58

with a sharp needle, "pinching skin and muscle" with forceps, exploration of the mouth with a probe, passive movement of the extremities, electric current, noise, light, water drops, etc. Such a battery of methods of stimulation has rarely been used on any organism. Local muscle contractions were secured at 27 days of copulation age to faradic current stimulation, before any spontaneous movements (28 days) were executed and before responses to exteroceptive stimulation could be secured at 31 days.

The sequence of spontaneous movements executed by

the embryos *in amnio* between 28 and 31 postcopulation days has close similarity to that for reactive behavior as described by Pankratz for the rabbit and Angulo for the rat. Carmichael's sequence for exteroceptive responses is divided into five stages, in the first of which "certain aspects of what will later form the typical 'pattern' of the gross responses from that area are released. By 'gross responses' is meant large limb-muscle and trunk movements" (1934, p. 430). However, he found that limbs moved at an early time toward the area stimulated, in conjunction with other bodily movements. This is an almost unique finding and is difficult to understand, as early movements have seldom been observed to have an apparently adaptive application of this sort. Most investigators have described the early trunk movements as being of a type that is of the nature of an avoiding response, although there are exceptions, as will be noted shortly.

In Carmichael's second stage the "pattern of gross movement which appeared weakly and incompletely in Stage A is now stronger and in many cases more 'adaptive,' " and specific reflexes begin to appear in his third stage. In the fourth stage, the "larger pattern" has become less complete with the increase in the "local responses" although it "can still be evoked." In his fifth stage, previously effective receptor areas tend to produce only "fast and precisely localized" responses or previously distinct patterns of reactivity tend to merge into newer and larger patterns of the entire organism. Carmichael has been contra-Coghillian in viewpoint because he believed the earlier exteroceptive responses to be far more complex in character than described by Coghill.

Carmichael was kind enough to demonstrate to me

one of the relatively early responses of the guinea-pig embryos. A stiff bristle was inserted into the external auditory canal, the region regarded by Carmichael as the first sensitive skin area in the guinea pig. A marked adduction movement of the ipsilateral forelimb resulted, accompanied by a slight neck flexion. It is easy to attribute responses to what some investigators, myself included, would regard as abnormally stiff or sharp stimulators, but the human embryo, the only mammalian form with which I have had extensive personal experience, does not respond to any stimulation in this area at a comparable stage of development. Except for these peculiar and unique movements, which may be a species difference, the sequence as worked out by Carmichael for the guinea pig has greater resemblance to the total pattern than to the additive idea originally put forward by Swenson. It is also true that the apparent greater complexity of early movements may be a matter of interpretation based upon the greater early participation of the forelimbs in mammals, in particular, than in amphibians. It is certain that adduction of the forelimbs occurs earlier in the guinea pig than it does in the human embryo and this may well be the basis of their "adaptive" movement toward the site of stimulation.

Bridgman and Carmichael (1935) found that responses to electrical stimulation preceded other types of activity which they regarded as reflexes. Slightly later (at 622 hours), the early guinea-pig fetuses responded to stimulation of the intact amniotic sac, either by exertion of pressure on it or by lightly striking its surface, by independent head or forelimb movements. Some 10 to 14 hours later, spontaneous movements of the same type appeared. Lateral trunk flexion often with neck flexion to form a C-type response, though at other times independently, could be elicited at 643 hours. These investigators believe that independent movements of a reflex nature occur at all times even in 712-hour fetuses, the oldest re-examined by them in this study.

Discussion now turns to the work of Windle and his associates (1930-1950). It is this group which ultimately espoused Swenson's idea of the origin of mammalian embryonic reactivity by the successive addition of "simple" reflexes. However, Windle and Griffin (1931), in their studies on spontaneous and reactive movements in the cat embryo, reported a sequence very close to Coghillian in its characteristics (table 4).

An element of doubt concerning the correctness of these earlier results began to appear in the 1933 paper by Windle, O'Donnell, and Glasshagle, which was also on the cat embryo. The earliest spontaneous movements observed at 24 days were first in the forelimb, later in the neck. However, they still considered the "mass movements" of the head, neck, and limbs to be totally integrated from the beginning. Tapping of the amnion and stimulation with a fine steel needle or a cactus thorn were the methods used. Both needle and thorn might be considered ill adapted to avoidance of direct mechanical stimulation. Some of their statements are of interest in this connection: "Simple, local, unit muscular contractions can be elicited a day earlier than spontaneous mass movements," but these may not be reflexes; localized stimulation elicited "isolated movements locally and reflex contractions of muscles in regions rostrad. However, reflexes farther caudad never ensue until after the expanding massive total pattern (locomotor re-

TABLE 4

Table of activities of the cat fetus, from Windle and Griffin, 1931. (By permission of the Wistar Institute of Anatomy and Biology.)

	Length of specimens (C R in mm.)	14	16	17	17.5	18.5	19.5–20	21–22	22.5	26	27–28	36	38	45	50	50–54	58–60	75–80	95–103	110	135–140
	Copulation age of specimens	23	24+	24.5	?	?	25	26	27	28	30	31	33	35	36	?	?	42	?	?	?
INTRINSIC HEAD MUSCLES	Laryngeal muscles (phonation)																—	—	+	+	+
	Facial muscles											—	—	—	—	—	±	—	+	+	+
	Tongue muscles										—	?	—	±	±		+	+	+	+	+
	Masticator muscles										+	+	+	+	+	+	+	+	+	+	+
HIND LIMB	Flexion of digits																—	?	+	+	+
	Adduction of limb														—	—	?	?	+	+	+
	Flexion at the ankle											—	—	—	?	?	+	+	+	+	+
	Flexion at the knee									—	—	±	+	+	+	+	+	+	+	+	+
	Flexion at hip							—	—	+	+	+	+	+	+	+	+	+	+	+	+
	Movement of pelvis (trunk)							+	+	+	+	+	+	+	+	+	+	+	+	+	+
FORE LIMB	Flexion of digits											—	—	—	?	—	?	+	+	+	+
	Adduction of limb							—	—	—	—	?	+	+	+	+	+	+	+	+	+
	Flexion at wrist							?	—	—	+	±	+	+	+	+	+	+	+	+	+
	Flexion at elbow						—	—	+	+	+	+	+	+	+	+	+	+	+	+	+
	Active flexion at shoulder (total flexion)		—	—	—	?	+	+	+	+	+	+	+	+	+	+	+	+	+	+	+
	'Passive' flexion at shoulder (total flexion)			+	+	+	+	+	+	+	+	+	+								
NECK AND TRUNK	Diaphragm											—	—	—	—	?	?	+	+	+	+
	Intercostal muscles											±	?	?	+	+	+	+	+	+	+
	Abdominal muscles											±	?	?	+	+	+	+	+	+	+
	Flexion of tail							—	—	—	—	±	+	+	+	+	+	+	+	+	+
	Rotation of trunk						—	+	+	+	+	+	+	+	+	+	+	+	+	+	+
	Flexion (ventral) of lower trunk				—	—	+	+	+	+	+	+	+	+	+	+	+	+	+	+	+
	Rotation of head			—	?	+	+	+	+	+	+	+	+	+	+	+	+	+	+	+	+
	Bilateral flexion of head and upper trunk		—	—	—	+	+	+	+	+	+	+	+	+	+	+	+	+	+	+	+
	Unilateral / Ventral flexion of head and upper trunk	—	+	+	? + ?	+ +	+ +	+ +	+ +	+ +	+ +	+ +	+ +	+ +	+ +	+ +	+ +	+ +	+ +	+ +	+ +

action) has extended below the points stimulated" (p. 540).

Windle, Orr, and Minear (1934), in their further studies on cat embryos, found that direct muscle stimulation could cause contractions at 23 days of copulation age and that the first reflexes appeared in some cases on the 24th day. Furthermore, limb movements followed 'pressure" stimuli earlier than they could be elicited by faradic shocks or by touch, but the reverse was true of head extension.

In his 1934 paper, again on cat embryos, Windle (1934b) made known his complete reversal to the "simple" reflex idea in the following statements: "Morphologically and physiologically, there is no evidence that the concept of a gradually expanding total pattern completely integrated from the beginning (Coghill, '29) can be applied to the first leg reflexes of the cat embryo. A series of unisegmental reflex arcs has been demonstrated at the time reflexes appear. The location of these in the upper brachial segments is correlated with the physiological observations. . . . Of course the local reflex arcs must eventually be integrated with each other as well as with more distant centers in the central nervous system" (1934*b*, pp. 501-502). These items will be discussed later in some detail.

Windle now turned his attention to an attempt to assay the effects of removal of cat embryos from the uterus in an effort to determine the "behavioral capabilities" of embryos after delivery, which are manifestly not those obtaining in the normal intra-uterine environment. This was begun in a communication by Windle, Minear, Austin, and Orr (1935). Nonmotile stage embryos were subjected to faradic stimulation. Under such stimulation, as these authors pointed out, the responses were always maximal and without latent period. The muscle tissue was held in a tetanic stage during the shock and relaxed slowly when it ceased. There was no refractory period, contractions being obtainable at will. The response was always localized and depended on the position of the electrodes. Furthermore, the physiological state of the embryo was without effect, the responses secured from dying or recently dead embryos being of the same character and elicited with the same facility as from those freshly exposed.

Attention was then turned to reflex behavior, and the time of eliciting the first reflexes was advanced from the previously stated time of 24 days to the 16th day. The methods of stimulation were "flipping" of the forelimb or tapping the embryo or amnion. Limb "flipping" or snout tapping caused movements of the limb or head, respectively, the former usually being independent of trunk movements. Each of the qualities of responses secured by the means mentioned were the exact opposite of those obtained by faradic current, viz., they were quick, nonmaximal, with definite latent and refractory periods, nontetanic, stereotyped without relation to the site of stimulation, and elicitable only from freshly exposed embryos. An interesting note is that "all reflexes seemed to require strong stimuli administered over relatively large areas in their incipiency" (p. 174). The question of strength of stimuli required for early reflexes is another aspect to be considered later.

In 1936, after having worked in Sir Joseph Barcroft's laboratory at Cambridge University, where sheep embryos were being studied, Windle published a short article on the activities of this and other forms. He stated that the responses secured in response to forelimb "flipping" and tapping on the intact amnion were probably "local, isolated movements, independent of and not as yet incorporated into any behavior pattern; that each involves the nervous as well as the muscular system and probably more than one neurone. I suggest that these embryonic movements are essentially reflexes of an elementary sort. They should not be confused with myogenic contractions, from which they differ in a number of respects" (p. 32*P*). "I invite a consideration of the probability that mammalian somatic behavior has its genesis in simple, non-integrated, spinal type reflexes" (p. 33*P*).

From 1938 to 1942, Windle and his collaborators turned their attention to the subject of anoxemia and its effect upon embryonic activity. They developed, early in this study, the thesis that all activities of early embryos examined more than a minute or so after the opening of the uterus, whether or not the embryo was still attached to a normal placental circulation, were abnormal by reason of the hypoxic condition produced. In 1944, Windle's "synthesizing article" presented these concepts in some detail. Here he re-emphasized the rapidity with which hypoxia abolishes early limb reflexes and transforms the original homolateral responses to a contralateral type. He thus believed that all Coghillian type responses (contralateral total pattern responses) in mammals were due to the hypoxic or asphyxial conditions induced by opening the uterus.

The work of Windle and his associates has been presented in such detailed review because it represents the chief challenge to the work of so many others and because a number of his claims will be examined in the third chapter. He began with a more or less Coghillian view but gradually adopted Swenson's (1929) "simple" reflex additive concept and his limb-flip technique. He ended with the belief that the total pattern type of response was solely due to the anoxic state of the removed fetus. These beliefs are reiterated in his 1950 (1950*b*) paper.

From 1936 to 1950, Barcroft, chiefly with Barron, but also with others, and Barron studied intensively the development of motility in sheep embryos. Work on this form had been published prior to 1936, but, because of the use of anesthetics which affected the activities of the fetus, it will not be considered here.

In 1936, Windle worked in Barcroft's laboratory, as previously noted, and the paper published in that year by Barcroft, Barron, and Windle largely reflects the views of the third author. However, as Barcroft and Barron continued their studies, their results caused them gradually to shift in the direction of a Coghillian sequence, and in 1939 they stated: "So far therefore as local and mass responses are concerned in the sheep, local mechanisms do appear to become segrated out from the total response in the sense implied by Coghill in his account of the development of behavior in Amblystoma" (1939*b*, p. 500).

Barcroft and Barron (1939*a*, 1939*b*) have summarized their previous studies (1936, 1937) and noted the sequence of events in the sheep embryo (gestation period, 147 days). The first activities exhibited were "spontaneous," appearing on the 35th day in favorable cases and consisting of lateral flexions of the trunk and head, produced by contraction of the long back muscles, and accompanied by abduction of the "poorly developed" ipsilateral forelimb. The movements were quick in execution and in return to posture.

At 38 days, the trunk was still flexed laterally, but the head was now extended and both fore and hind limbs were abducted. These "spontaneously" executed movements occurred repeatedly, establishing a kind of rapid rhythm, from side to side. At the same time, movements of the liver appeared to indicate that the diaphragm was contracting as a part of the "generalized" activity, inasmuch as (1936) such diaphragmatic contractions could not be elicited at this time by asphyxial conditions.

Between 41 and 47 days, limb activity began on an increased tempo and amplitude, but associated with the movements of the trunk. Eye movements, as part of the "generalized" "spontaneous" activity, were observed on the 50th day. When the head was moved suddenly in a "clockwise" direction, the left eye was "just preceptibly" moved downward.

These "spontaneous" movements, increasing in extent and amplitude with age, were so called because no specific stimulus could be assigned as their cause. However, because these "spontaneous" movements tended to disappear if the uterus or amniotic sac were left undisturbed for a period and immediately to begin again if either were moved, Barcroft and Barron concluded that the movement of uterus or sac caused afferent neuron stimulation, at least in large part, if not entirely. They were unimpressed by the notion that such movements were caused by "accumulated metabolites, principally CO_2," as they were never able to produce these movements by inducing asphyxial conditions at this age.

In studying induced activity caused by faradic stimuli,

Barcroft and Barron attempted to apply the stimulus within areas supplied by known sensory nerves. They found that the area supplied by the maxillary division (V_2) of the trigeminal nerve became sensitive at 34 days, especially in the region below the eye. Faradic stimulation in this area caused rotation of the occiput away from the stimulator and contralateral flexion of the neck, a movement which caused the snout to approach the electrodes. Sometimes movement of the ispilateral forelimb followed or accompanied the head movement and, in somewhat older fetuses, this movement of the forelimb became a constant component of the response.

By 38 days, faradic stimulation over the infraorbital foramen caused contralateral rotation of the occiput, forelimb extension and extension of the trunk and tail, the hind limbs moving only passively with the trunk extension. By 40 days, this series of action components was accompanied by opening of the mouth, seen only occasionally at 38 days. At 40 days also, touching a thin glass rod to the tip of the snout caused head and trunk extension, bilateral forelimb extension and pelvic flexion, as a result of stimulation of V_2 on both sides at once. When only one V_2 area was so stimulated, however, head rotation to the ipsilateral side, ipsilateral trunk flexion, extension and partial abduction of the homolateral, and flexion of the contralateral, forelimb, with either flexion or extension of the hind limbs, resulted. These two types of activity were clearly initiated by the trunk musculature and its maintenance of the response posture lasted longer than that of head or limbs.

Various other nerve areas were also tested. Glass-rod stimulation of the tongue caused only mouth closure at 42 days, but by 59 days evidence of sucking was observed.

In addition, chewing and swallowing activities were seen to accompany the sucking movements by 80 days.

The area supplied by the mandibular division (V_3) of the trigeminal was markedly retarded over V_2 in becoming sensitive to tactile stimulation. Only on the 50th day did glass rod stroking in the V_3 area cause a response, limited to opening of the mouth. By 60 days, the mouth opened and the head turned toward the rod.

The area supplied by the ophthalmic division (V_1) became sensitive earlier than the V_3 region, at 40 days. Responses to stimulation of this area were much the same as secured from V_2.

Other skin areas of the body do not become sensitive to stimulation with a fine glass rod before the 44th day and no "generalized" responses were secured elsewhere than in the facial region.

The studies of Barcroft and Barron, reviewed above quite incompletely, form one of the most carefully controlled investigations yet made on infrahuman mammals. They again emphasize that generic differences in the nature of the activity sequence occur, indeed are to be expected.

* * * * * *

The foregoing review of studies on the development of activity in the infrahuman vertebrate phylogenetic series demonstrates that two major points of view (and several minor ones) have been advanced in explanation of the fundamental nature of the behavioral sequence. One of the major concepts may be termed the Coghillian, the other the Windelian, for their respective principal proponents.

The Coghillian concept maintains that reactive behavior starts as a total pattern, in the sense that all of the neuromuscular mechanism which is capable of functioning participates from the beginning. This total pattern expands as more and more of the neuromuscular mechanism becomes functional. A necessary part of this development to the functional level of nerves and muscles in the normal cephalocaudal differentiation of the organism is the integration of the new neural elements with those that have already become functional. Such integration is a part of the morphological process of development and is completed before function of these new elements begins.

When the total pattern has been completed, specific, more or less local, reflexes ("partial patterns") first appear ("become individuated"). Such specific reflexes also tend to appear in a generally cephalocaudal and proximodistal direction. They are made possible by the further development of new neural elements which are likewise integrated into the total pre-existing functioning nervous mechanism before they can begin to participate in the expanding activity of the embryo. It would thus appear that these specific local reflexes are by no means unitary and simple, but are derived as a result of the increased complexity of the nervous system during its development.

The exact nature of activities which compose the developing behavioral sequence of any given animal form differs, at least in particulars, from that of any other. Nevertheless, the broad concept of an expanding total pattern from which specific local activities are secondarily derived seems to hold throughout the vertebrates.

The second major viewpoint, originated by Swenson but receiving its major support from the conclusions of Windle, is based on an almost diametrically opposed concept. Windle has denied that there is any thread of basic similarity running throughout the vertebrate ontogenetic series. He states that Coghill's concept applies only to amphibian forms. In the mammals, Windle has claimed that behavior develops by the appearance of a localized, non-integrated, unitary response, then, seriatim, of others which become secondarily integrated with those pre-existing. In the birds, he believes the activity may be intermediate between the total pattern and unitary types of reflexes, resulting in an admixture leading preponderantly toward the latter concept.

In addition, Windle has stated that the mammalian unit reflexes, described by him, are elicitable only during an extremely short period of time, measurable in seconds rather than minutes, and only under the most favorable conditions. Manipulation of the uterus or of the fetus alters the normal O_2-CO_2 content of the fetal blood almost instantly and induces relatively immediate anoxia or asphyxia. In consequence, responses secured after the first moments of exposure are abnormal, in his view, their abnormality being due to anoxia. This concept of the method of origin of overt behavior in the mammals is extended by Windle to that of man, to be considered in the next chapter. Following consideration of the varying views concerning the development of embryonic and fetal behavior in man, the two major basic concepts will be further discussed in the last chapter.[5]

Chapter 2

The Sequence in Human Fetal Activity

IT HAS PROVED a difficult task to determine the number of human embryos or fetuses the early activity of which has been described by scientific observers only, and it is impossible to give any data regarding the very early statements of those non-scientists who have observed them. Inasmuch as even the earlier observers with some scientific affiliations gave only casual notes of quite uncontrolled examinations, a complete list of references to them can have only historical interest. Although Erbkam (1837) appears to be the first scientist to record observations of a living human fetus, to be followed by Pflüger (1877), Zuntz (1877), Rawitz (1879), Preyer (1885), Strassman (1903), Yanase (1907), Krabbe (1912), Winterstein (1914), Bersot (1920-1921), Woyciechowski (1928), Liesch (1946), Davis and Potter (1946), Langreder (1949), and Barcroft (unpublished), adequately controlled studies did not begin to appear until about 1920, with the first publication of Minkowski.

Minkowski's studies (1920-1946) covered some 75 or more fetuses and constitute the classic fundamental contribution on the subject. His work on the development of the plantar reflex (1923, 1926) bids fair to retain its validity for a long time to come. Nevertheless, Minkowski's interpretations were those of a psychiatrist relatively untrained in embryology. In consequence, the earlier activities observed by him are open to other interpretations.

His observed facts are unexpectedly accurate in view of the complex movements exhibited by young human fetuses and the rapidity with which they are executed, for Minkowski did not have the advantage of objective motion-picture recording of the activities observed. To observe, analyze, and record movements as they occur requires a master observer and this Minkowski has proved himself to be.

In 1924, Bolaffio and Artom published the results of their observations on some 28 human fetuses, insofar as they can be identified as separate cases. Unlike Minkowski, these investigators exercised little effort to maintain a normal condition of the fetuses during their observations and the methods of stimulation used were not well adapted to the problem. Their results, therefore, cannot be evaluated satisfactorily.

These were the only two studies of any magnitude when the group in the Department of Anatomy at the University of Pittsburgh School of Medicine began, in 1932, the studies which will be discussed later in this chapter. However, in 1937, Windle and Fitzgerald published their first paper on seven human embryos 7 to 8 weeks of age, none of which moved. Later, Fitzgerald and Windle (1942) described the activities of four of their total of 17 embryos observed to that time and these findings deserve detailed presentation.

Two of Fitzgerald and Windle's four active embryos were observed while the placental connections and amnion were intact and within a very short time after exposure by a uterine incision. These two embryos were, respectively, 22.5 mm. (7½ weeks) and 23 mm. (stated to be 8 weeks) in crown-rump (CR) length. In the smaller of these, the authors believed that anoxemia had already begun, as no movements resulted from tapping on the amnion. However, "strong" stimulation with a needle in the mouth region caused a contralateral flexion of the trunk. On still stronger stimulation, the arms and legs moved with the trunk in the resulting flexion. Only pressure produced responses, no reflexes being secured by touch or stroking. Although homolateral flexions of the trunk were more numerous, contralateral flexions were observed. Pinching or heavy stroking of the trunk or limbs caused "contractions of the muscles in the immediate vicinity" (p. 162).

When the amnion of the 23 mm. embryo was tapped "so lightly that the fetus within was scarcely jarred," "quick reactions of the limbs or lower trunk" occurred. The "arms or legs moved sharply caudad" (p. 162) at times and once the trunk flexed ventrally. Stronger tapping on the amnion caused simultaneous movements of all appendages.

The other two fetuses were 20 mm. and 26 mm. in CR length. In both, the placenta had just separated from the endometrium. In the 20 mm. embryo (7½ weeks), no reflexes were observed on the operating table, but a minute after placental separation, while it was in Locke's solution, "strong" mechanical stimulation in the maxillary area caused definite contralateral flexion of the trunk, without participation of either arms or legs.

When the amnion of the 26 mm. CR (8½ weeks) embryo was tapped, the arms and legs responded as they had in the 23 mm. embryo, but these movements were accompanied by lateral flexion of the head and trunk. Fitzgerald and Windle believe that anoxia was developing in this specimen, since the embryo was "less excitable" than the 23 mm. case.

* * * * * *

The Pittsburgh studies on the physiological responses of human embryos and fetuses were begun in 1932 by the writer (1936-1944). Morphological studies on the physiologically tested cases incapable of survival were started almost immediately by Dr. Ira D. Hogg and are being continued by Dr. Tryphena Humphrey. Some of the results of the morphological work will be presented in the third chapter, but the remainder of this chapter will be devoted to the sequence of fetal activity as shown by the physiological studies. However, it seems advisable first to review the factors which might modify the validity of the results secured and the measures taken to combat their effects.

In general, it may be said that three types of factors must be overcome, insofar as it is possible to do so: the progressive anoxic condition of the embryo, maternal anesthesia, and a group of physical factors. The progressive hypoxia of the embryo is, of course, produced by the placental separation that occurs within one to two and a half minutes before the initiation of stimulation. If the placenta, attached by the umbilical cord to the embryo, is placed under an atmosphere or more of oxygen in a separate container, it is possible to improve the fetal heart rate materially and to prolong the period during which it continues to beat. Both rate and amplitude of the heart beat may be altered at will by withholding or supplying oxygen. However, such administration of oxygen to the placenta has no discernible effect either upon the nature of the responses elicitable or upon the length of time during which they may be secured. This factor, then, must be endured, for the present at least, unless one may examine fetuses *in utero* as was done by Fitzgerald and Windle. Just how important or unimportant it may be during the earliest responses secured will be discussed later (pp. 102-110). Fetuses of about 23½ weeks or older may be resuscitated and, during the period of respiration, which increases with the age of the fetus, activities are entirely normal, as the hypoxic state is absent.

The second factor affecting the activity of the fetus is maternal anesthesia in those cases removed operatively. It has been our experience in Pittsburgh that the barbiturates (amytal, monosodium isoamyl, ethyl barbiturate, nembutal or pentobarbital sodium) rather completely anesthetize the fetus so that activity is eliminated. Injections of picrotoxin counteract barbiturate anesthesia, but its use in embryos and very young fetuses presents difficulties, if not abnormalities of motion, because of the volume it is necessary to inject. Coramine is another drug favored by some physicians to overcome anesthesia, but its effect is at least doubtful.

Other drugs tend to reduce fetal activity, but do not eliminate it, unless given the mother in massive amounts. Nevertheless, their use is considered in these studies as inimical to the observation of normal activity, although there will be further comment on this point (p. 109). Such drugs are avertin (tribromoethyl alcohol), ether, nitrous oxide, and morphine. The first two are more apt to eliminate fetal activity than the others.

Certain drugs, as novocaine and similar compounds, either locally or as spinal anesthetic, demerol (meperidine hydrochloride), atropin or ephedrin, when given the mother, appear to have no affect upon fetal activity. In consequence, when fetuses are secured by hysterotomy, we have gradually learned to use for this study only fetuses from cases where the attending obstetrician has decided to use local or spinal novocaine and where preoperative medication consists only of demerol, atropin, or ephedrine.

The physical factors which might affect the normal nature of the results are: release from intra-uterine pressures, disappearance of temperature control, and physical insults afforded by operative procedures or premature birth. Very little can be done about the release from intra-uterine pressures incident to removal of the embryo or fetus from the uterus by operation or by spontaneous premature birth. Actually, there is no difference between the activities of embryos observed within the intact amniotic sac, where the pressures differ perhaps little from those *in utero*, and after their release from it. Older fetuses gain a freedom of action of the extremities which is largely denied them within the confining uterine walls.

Temperature can be controlled as readily outside the uterus as within, except for the moment of transfer. We have used a large and carefully regulated constant temperature bath and have utilized "gold glass" in front of the photographic spotlights to prevent their heat from affecting the fluid. Embryos and all fetuses too young to respire are examined in physiological saline, Tyrode's solution, or some similar isotonic medium, kept at body temperature. Fetuses which have been resuscitated are examined in heated "premature beds" in rooms warmed to 85° F.

The most serious factor in its effect on the embryo or fetus is the manipulation of the membranes and fetus in hysterotomy. Observation of the operator's care in avoiding trauma and examination of the fetus can give a basis for estimation of the seriousness of the damage done. However careful the removal has been, there is some insult. Nevertheless, the few young fetuses known to have been damaged, as shown by multiple petechial hemorrhages under the skin, have often responded actively and in a manner indistinguishable from that of fetuses not so affected.

Two methods have been used to record the activities exhibited during the observations: motion pictures and dictated notes. Chief reliance has been placed upon the motion picture records, which permit exact and repeated analysis of the components of each response and are entirely objective in nature. Dictated notes are made to record activities which it was not certain had been "caught" by the motion picture camera. Such notes are rarely used in the study unless supported by the cinematographic record. Ordinarily, 35 mm. negative film is used for normal operation, but 16 mm. negative film has been used for "slow motion" recording and 16 mm. reversible film was employed during the war when 35 mm. was not available. All positive prints are made on 16 mm. film.

In the Pittsburgh studies 131 cases have been observed.[6] The fetuses range in age from 6½ weeks of menstrual age to a postmature of 45 weeks. It is interesting to note that four of the 131 cases were twins, but, with one exception, only one twin of each pair was studied intensively. Of the 131 cases observed, two failed to exhibit movement probably because they were too young (6½ weeks), 14 failed to show responses because of deep anesthesia or injury, and 31 moved, but their activities were possibly reduced or modified by the administration of anesthetic or hypnotic drugs to the mother. The remaining 84 were secured by hysterotomy or hysterectomy under novocaine spinal or local anesthesia or, in the cases of older fetuses, were born spontaneously without the use of drugs. These 84 and the two which were probably too young to move may be considered entirely unanesthetized. The report is based on the 84.

The standard method of stimulation employed to test for reflexes is stroking restricted areas of the skin with a hair. The hairs used are calibrated to provide maximum pressures of 10, 25, 50, 100 mg., 2 and 5 gm. The 10 mg. hairs are human; those capable of exerting greater pressures are horsehairs of carefully selected diameters. Each hair is mounted in a glass tube with hard paraffin and calibrated by the cut-and-test method. The mounting is held vertically over one pan of an accurate chainomatic balance, with the desired weight on the other side. Each hair is then cut until it keeps the pan on which it is pressed in exact balance with the weight when bent maximally but with only the tip of the hair touching the pan. The tip of the hair is then beaded with a tiny drop of inert liquid cement to prevent its cut end from abrading or penetrating the skin. When this has dried smoothly, the hair is retested to be certain its "pressure value" remains the same. Repeated tests have shown that the warm solution used for the embryo does not alter a hair's "pressure value" during the period of any observation.

As the full pressure of such a hair can only be exerted when it is forced down upon one point and as such "spot stimulation" is rarely an effective stimulus, the pressure exerted in the light stroke over the skin used to produce exteroceptive stimulation is far less than its "pressure value." Beaded glass rods for pressure stimulation and electric stimuli are also used, at times. Unless otherwise specified, the results given in the account which follows are from stimulation with a hair.

The determination of the age of a human embryo or fetus is very difficult. Many women, and especially those in a ward population, have only a hazy idea of the date of onset of the last menstrual period (L.M.P.). With some notable exceptions, patients will furnish a date—any date—for the L.M.P., when urged. Examination of the level of development of the embryo or fetus proves that little dependence can be placed upon the date given for that particular L.M.P. In consequence, some other means of staging embryos and fetuses by age must be used. There are innumerable formulas and tables for determining age from length. Only two seem to have value. The tables published by the late George L. Streeter in 1920 were used in these studies, partly because they were the only reliable ones available when these studies were begun and partly because experience has indicated that they fit the Pittsburgh population well. In 1941, Edith Boyd published formulas and curves for age determination based on both crown-rump and crown-heel length. Boyd used a wide range of data, some from Minnesota and some from other regions. Her tables are probably more scientifically validated than Streeter's, but we have continued to adhere to our original staging. Furthermore, we have used menstrual age throughout, as attempts to "correct" it to "actual" age merely confound confusion.

* * * * * *

Until about the middle of the 7th week of menstrual age, the human embryo appears to be incapable of any type of reflex activity. There is certainly no area of integument sensitive to exteroceptive stimulation before this time. The musculature of the human embryo may be electrically stimulated to contraction beginning with the latter part of the 6th week, but contractions so produced are sharply localized at this or at any subsequent age. There appears to be no true myogenic activity in human embryos.

From approximately the middle of the 7th to just before the 8th week, when the embryo is between 20 and 23 mm. CR, stimulation by lightly stroking the upper or lower lip or the alae of the nose with a hair exerting a maximum bending pressure of 10 or 25 mg. causes typically a contralateral flexion of the neck and uppermost trunk, with little or no participation of the upper extremities and none of any other portion of the body. Two such cases have been observed in the Pittsburgh studies. From one (93A, 20.7 mm. CR), only a single response without visible participation of the upper extremities was elicited. From the other (No. 131, 22.6 mm. CR), a large number of identical responses was secured. In these the upper extremities quivered slightly during the contralateral neck and upper trunk flexion, as though its musculature were attempting to contract. This quivering motion extended even to the fingers, but the upper extremities did not move otherwise. The skin area sensitive to stimulation was limited to the region immediately about the mouth. Although previously it was believed that some slightly older embryos (8+ to 8½ weeks) showed sensitivity in the area supplied by the maxillary division of the fifth cranial nerve a shade earlier than in that supplied by the mandibular division, this was not confirmed in either of the embryos here described.

To these two cases from the Pittsburgh series may be

added the two, previously described, which were observed by Fitzgerald and Windle (1942). Their 20 mm. embryo, showing no responses on the operating table, gave definite contralateral flexions of the "trunk," without arm movement, following "strong" mechanical stimulation of the maxillary region. Their 22.5 mm. embryo, also showing no movements on tapping of the amnion, exhibited both ipsilateral and contralateral flexions of the trunk, both arms and legs moving with the trunk, on stimulation with a needle in the mouth region. The latter embryo responded more like one of 8½ weeks and was, in fact, estimated by them at 8 weeks of age.

There is no active or unanesthetized embryo of exactly 8 weeks in the Pittsburgh series, but there are six embryos of 8½ weeks (25 to 28 mm. CR) which moved, one of which is subject to suspicion of being possibly slightly anesthetized because morphine had been administered to the mother. The five unanesthetized cases all responded to unilateral exteroceptive stimulation in the mouth region by light stroking with a hair, and the responses were, in each case, practically identical with every other when repeated. They were, thus, stereotyped.

The typical response at 8½ weeks consists of the following elements: 1) chiefly contralateral flexion of the neck and trunk, though two ipsilateral flexions are recorded; 2) extension (backward movement) of the arms at the shoulder, without participation of the elbow, wrist, or fingers; 3) rotation of the pelvis toward the contralateral side, with no noticeable independent participation of the lower extremities. The neck-trunk flexion and the arm extension were simultaneous. The pelvic (rump) rotation, slight in the younger embryos, occurs with the trunk flexion in these younger cases but tends to have an extremely short period of delay in those of increasing length (and, presumably, older) when the rotation has become somewhat more pronounced.

The relaxation of the movement (return to posture) is accomplished first by the arms, then by the neck, trunk, and rump, which tend to hold their flexion-rotation posture momentarily. Because the body of the embryo rolls as a result of the trunk flexion, return to the exact position occupied before the response does not always occur. However, the difference is slight. A series of such responses may be elicited at short intervals for as long as three to four minutes after beginning placental separation. Each response is, within relatively minute biological variations, identical with every other, hence these responses are also stereotyped. However, as the time interval between the response and beginning placental separation lengthens and the degree of anoxia increases, the threshold rises gradually, requiring increasingly higher "pressure value" hairs to evoke a response.

As the young fetus approaches the 9½-week age, centering around 34 mm. CR, the rump rotation becomes still more marked and tends to become separated from the usually contralateral trunk flexion and bilateral arm extension at the shoulder as a distinct phase of the response. Although the vigor of movement of the caudal end of the trunk has increased over that seen at 8½ weeks, the skin area sensitive to stimulation remains the same. Furthermore, spontaneously executed movements in the form of the typical response first to one side, then to the other, are clearly evident at 9 to 9½ weeks, but only for a very short time, limited to about one minute after the beginning of placental separation.

There is some evidence that such spontaneously executed activity might be present at 8½ weeks. One 8½-week embryo (No. 116, 27.1 mm. CR) reacted repeatedly to stimulation in the sensitive area by side-to-side repetitions of the typical response. Another (No. 24, 26 mm. CR) gave a single contralateral-ipsilateral response to perioral stimulation a few minutes after delivery. These instances were in response to definite exteroceptive stimulation, but were of the bilateral nature typical of spontaneous activities. The similar, but truly spontaneous, movements seen at 9 to 9½ weeks were not in response to identifiable external stimulation.

At 9½ weeks, another method of exciting the typical response, consisting of lateral trunk flexion, bilateral arm extension, and rump rotation, was accidentally discovered. To center a fetus (No. 16) under the lens, it was rapidly rotated by the umbilical attachment of the membranes without any contact being made with the usual reflexogenic perioral area. A very complete typical response resulted. This was formerly (1944 *et ante*) interpreted as a vestibular response. It is absent in two 8½-week fetuses which were similarly rotated. So far as may be determined histologically, the vestibular apparatus appears complete at 9½ weeks. However, there is much evidence that vestibular function does not appear in cat or sheep until much later. Windle and Fish (1932), on the basis of their rotatory experiments with cat fetuses and ablation of the vestibular apparatus, present evidence that the vestibular righting reflex in this form does not appear earlier than the 54th day of gestation, although body-righting reflexes appear on the 50th day. Barcroft and Barron (1937, 1939*b*) state that vestibular responses do not appear in the sheep until the 43rd day after birth, although the "neck righting reflex," as they term it, can be evoked by the 50th day of gestation. In consequence, the post-rotation response in the human fetus would appear to be a body-righting reflex caused by the disturbance of head-body relations. However, Minkowski (1936) states that both "cervical tonic" and "labyrinthine" reflexes appear in the human fetus during the fourth month. This age is, of course, far greater than that of the 9½-week fetus in which the response under discussion was found.

At the 9½-week level, passive extension of the fingers has caused flexion at the wrist, elbow, and shoulder. These appear to be typical stretch responses, proprioceptive in nature.

If the description so far given of responses from about 7½ to 9½ weeks has accomplished its purpose, it should be evident that the earliest responses secured were flexion, predominantly contralateral, of neck and upper trunk without participation of the extremities. This was followed by more complete trunk flexion with extension of both upper extremities at the shoulder-joint and a slight pelvic or rump rotation, without movement of the lower extremities as such. Next in turn came marked lateral flexion of the trunk, preponderantly contralateral, bilateral arm extension, and such complete rump rotation that the lower extremities appeared to participate, especially so in the body-righting response. Except for a short period around 8 weeks, every step in the caudal progression of the response has been observed. During the period from 7½ to about 10 weeks, the only skin area sensitive to a light stroking with a hair is limited to the perioral distribution of the maxillary and mandibular divisions of the fifth cranial nerve. These early responses would appear to constitute a continually expanding total pattern. No other explanation fits the observed phenomena.

From 9½ to 10½ weeks there is no change in the nature of the response to stimulation in the perioral region. At about 10½ weeks the palms of the hands become sensitive to strokes with a light hair, partial closure of the fingers resulting. In the finger-closing response, the thumb frequently does not participate. Three to five days later, stimulation of the volar or lateral surfaces of the upper arm may cause independent arm extension at the shoulder; of the upper eyelid, contraction of the orbicularis oculi muscle; and of the sole of the foot, plantar flexion of the toes. These responses have so far appeared in the order given, although independent arm extension has only rarely been seen. It will become apparent that it is easier to evoke responses from fingers or toes than from brachia, forearms, thighs, or legs.

At about 11 weeks, the previously typical response to perioral stimulation becomes modified by the appearance of an element of trunk extension, either alternating with or partially combined with the lateral flexion. Arm extension, which has hitherto accompanied the trunk flexion, is giving way to medial rotation of the brachia, which will reach its full development in another few days. There is also some slight rotation of the thighs in the total pattern response. Finger closure, still only partial and seldom accompanied by thumb flexion, follows palmar stimulation. Stimulation of the skin of the forearm may occasionally cause forearm pronation. Plantar flexion of the toes, with or without participation of the hallux, follows stimulation of the sole of the foot. Contraction of the orbicularis oculi and of the corrugator muscles may be elicited by stimulation either of the upper eyelid or of the eyebrow region of the forehead.

It will be noticed that the skin area sensitive to stimuli has been expanding. No longer limited to the perioral region, it now includes all skin over the front of the face and the whole of the upper and lower extremities. However, stimulation of the region innervated by the maxillary and mandibular divisions of V gives rise to total pattern type activity, of other areas to local responses only. On the trunk, there is no sensitive skin evident at 11 weeks. Only light stimuli are necessary to evoke responses over the face, hands, and feet, and the fetuses are active in responding. The total pattern type of response is thus modified by the appearance of a number of specific responses.

At 11½ weeks, the reflexogenous zone (area sensitive to stimuli) gives evidence of spreading downward over the upper chest. At this age, activities already present have become further perfected and additional new ones appear. Extension of the trunk is increasingly, but by no means entirely, replacing the hitherto typical lateral flexion. Trunk extension is especially marked when stimulation is in the midline of the face, but also occurs on stimulation elsewhere on the face. As one approaches closer to the end of the period during which reflexes can be elicited from an individual specimen, the lateral flexion type of response tends to increase in incidence, probably because of increasing asphyxia, although the locus of stimulation plays an important role. At this age, the medial rotation of the brachia accompanying the trunk movement has increased to the point where the two hands approach one another, although only the fingers touch. Rotation of the face to the opposite side has appeared in response to stimulation of the side of the face, but midline facial stimulation causes head extension. Head rotation is usually accompanied by lateral trunk flexion, head extension by trunk extension, and it is with the latter type of response that the medial rotation of the brachia reaches its maximum. Arm abduction or wrist or forearm flexion may follow stimulation of various areas of the skin of the upper extremity. Stimulation of the sole of the foot causes plantar flexion of the toes, flexion of the knee and thigh, and then a quick knee extension, resulting in a kick.

By 12 to 12½ weeks, the reflexogenous areas of the skin have not appreciably increased, but unilateral facial stimulation in the perioral region causes marked extension of neck and trunk accompanied by a wide variety of movements at many of the joints in the upper extremities. The responses are still quite mechanical in their execution and the fetuses continue to be very active, but there is somewhat greater variety in the exact components of the responses, one differing from another in the accompanying movements. The general response may be evoked by stimulation of either the region supplied by the maxillary division of the fifth cranial nerve (V_2) or that to which the mandibular division (V_3) passes. On one occasion, when V_3 had been stimulated, a contraction of the orbicularis oculi muscle of the same side was observed. Perioral stimulation has also caused, as activities accompanying the total pattern, such movements as: rapid contralateral elbow extension, then its flexion; lateral, then medial rotation of contralateral arm; and elevation of the shoulders.

At this age there are several specific reflexes which may be evoked. In at least two cases, stimulation over one eyelid was accompanied by a downward rotation of the eyeballs, made evident by the shift in the highlights on the still fused lids. Lip closure follows stimulation of the lips and, when repeated, may result in swallowing. Digital closure is incomplete but is usually accompanied by wrist flexion or a combined flexion-abduction motion. In 12½-week specimens, stimulation of the sole of the foot may result in dorsiflexion of the hallux and toe-fanning, or in plantar flexion of hallux and toes, though flexion of the hallux is likely to be less complete than that of the other digits, if not entirely absent.

By 12½ weeks, in the majority of cases, the total pattern activity is rapidly fading, being replaced by an increasing number of specific reflexes. Coghill, himself, has called these "partial patterns." Within the next ten days, the total pattern has almost completely disappeared, to be evoked only by extremes of stimulation. Some human fetuses have reached this stage by 13 weeks of menstrual age. Others at presumably the same age level still exhibit a stereotyped total pattern. All below the age of 13½ to 14 weeks tend to return to a total pattern type of response before asphyxia and other causes blot out further activity.

Specifically, at 13 weeks, unilateral stimulation in the perioral region may result in any one of the following response types, in addition to a total pattern shown by a few: 1) ipsilateral arm extension, only; 2) flexion of the head, bilateral arm extension, and extension of the ipsilateral thigh; 3) head extension, contralateral arm extension, and ipsilateral thigh flexion, knee extension, and dorsiflexion of the foot; 4) trunk and neck extension, rotating into a contralateral trunk flexion, without extremity participation; 5) contralateral turning of the face and flexion of the head away from the stimulus; or 6) turning of the face toward the stimulus. Stimulation over the extremities with hairs having pressure values of from 25 to 100 mg. or of 2 gm., depending on the degree of anoxia, may result in purely local responses of the part touched or of the entire extremity. This incomplete listing of responses exhibited serves to illustrate the transition from total pattern with some specific reflexes to a manifestation of specific responses almost solely, found between 13 and 14 weeks.

By 13½ to 14 weeks, except for the back and top of the head, almost the entire surface of the body is sensitive to stroking with a light hair. As noted, the total pattern type of response has practically disappeared. Unilateral stimulation of the face causes contralateral turning of the face alone, an avoiding response, accompanied by elevation of the angle of the mouth and nasal ala on the same side, if the hair touches the side of the nose, or a contraction of the orbicularis oculi muscle, if the stimulus is applied over the eyelids. If the lips only are stimulated, they are pressed together, without head rotation. Touching the inside of the lips or mouth may cause tongue movements. Swallowing sometimes follows lip stimulation, but usually only on repetition of the stimulus. Finger closure is complete, the pollex rarely entering into the formation of the resulting "fist," but the closure is relatively momentary, there being no sustained grasping response as yet. The quality of the responses is altered. Instead of the mechanical, stereotyped movement seen earlier, the various activities are graceful and "flowing." The fetus is very active.

The 13½- to 14-week period is an important one in the

development of human fetal activity. During the period of 6 to 6½ weeks after exteroceptive responses began as a total pattern at about 7½ weeks, many of the specific reflexes of the neonate have appeared, replacing the total pattern which has practically ceased to exist as such. Those reflexes which have made their appearance are concerned primarily with trunk, extremities, head, and face. They are not all in the final form they will assume, but, with the addition of a number not yet present, they lay the framework for gradual development into the reflexes of postnatal life. Among those reflexes which have not as yet appeared are, primarily, grasp, respiration, and phonation (the latter being of course dependent on the former), the suctorial reflex, and the tendon reflexes. Furthermore, the fetal muscles are weak and ineffective. In the remaining weeks of the gestation period, the increase in volume and strength of the muscles, the development of additional neuromuscular mechanism, and the growth of the lungs will occur.

During the remaining period of gestation, there will be almost no change in the sensitive areas of the body, as the back and top of the head remain relatively incapable of evoking reflexes for some time to come. There will, however, be a marked maturation of already existing reflexes and certain ones, now absent and probably requiring new central and neuromuscular connections, will gradually emerge.

By 15 weeks, there is definite evidence of maintained finger closure, sometimes, though rarely, noticeable several days earlier. This is the first appearance of grasping. At this time also the abdominal muscles are capable of sufficient contraction to provide a feeble sort of abdominal reflex when the stimulating hair is drawn across them. The fetus is active and the pre-existing reflexes are already becoming more vigorous as muscle maturation proceeds.

About a week later, the fetus begins to undergo a profound change in its reactivity. Periods of sluggishness tend to alternate with bursts of activity and the threshold for stimulation has increased. As age progresses, the periods of relative inactivity of the fetus become more prolonged and the bursts of activity more difficult to evoke. This is characteristic of the period beginning at about 17 to 18 weeks and continuing until the fetus may be caused to breathe at about 23½ weeks. Barcroft and Barron (1937) observed the same thing in sheep fetuses with intact placental connections. The cause is still undetermined. In the human fetuses observed, in which the placental connections had been interrupted, it is possible that the sluggishness may be due to accumulations of CO_2 which are eliminated by the ventilation of the lungs on resuscitation. Certain it is that the establishment of respiration soon abolishes any such sluggishness.

By 17 weeks, stimulation of the upper lip causes its protrusion. Similar gentle stroking of the lower lip at this age produces lip closure, as was the case with either lip at 12½ weeks.

Gasping, as a terminal agonal phenomenon without external stimulation, has been observed in fetuses as young as 13 weeks. This is accompanied by chest contractions, indicative of respiratory attempts, albeit ineffectual in causing breathing. By 18½ weeks, weak chest contractions, later to be accompanied by abdominal contractions and expansions, the latter proving diaphragmatic activity, have been observed in some cases in response to chest stimulation, or spontaneously, though these also are ineffectual in causing respiration. The earliest Pittsburgh case in which effective respiration, self-sustained for a brief period when once initiated, was observed was 23½ weeks old, as just noted. At 18½ weeks also, weakly effective grasping is present. A thin, moist glass rod laid in the palm will be held by maintained finger closure, so that it is possible to draw the arm across the chest by pulling the stimulator in the direction of its long axis. The thumb is not constantly involved in this primitive grasping. The fetus is notably sluggish in responding at this age. However, when reflexes are elicited by 100 mg. or 2 gm. hairs, the activity is vigorous.

By 20 weeks, stimulation of either upper or lower lip causes its protrusion and by 22 weeks there is definite pursing of the lips as well as protrusion. This is a preliminary step in the development of the suctorial response, but no actual suction is exerted as yet.

Between 18½ and 23½ weeks, the chest and abdominal contractions and expansions increase in incidence and amplitude, until brief but effective respiration, especially after use of the respirator, occurs. It may be that some fetuses younger than 23½ weeks might be resuscitated, but so far it has not been possible in this series. Whenever respiration occurs, phonation—only a high-pitched cry, of course—accompanies its initiation and may be repeated at intervals following the establishment of breathing. The establishment of respiration for 20 minutes or more completely abolishes the sluggish nature of the fetus. As its color begins to improve, for most fetuses of this age have at first a slightly cyanotic appearance even with intact placental connections, the fetus becomes more active than at any time heretofore. The arms and legs are very actively moved in all direction, the trunk is flexed and extended in all planes and it becomes possible to elicit various tendon reflexes—ankle clonus, knee jerk, etc.—not hitherto obtainable. The change in activity following respiration is startling, although, except for the possibility of eliciting tendon reflexes, no new activities appear. Indeed, little new appears during the next two or three weeks. It is almost as though the fetus were developing its respiratory capacity at the expense of the appearance of other new responses. This may, at least in part, be the result of the explosive appearance of "spontaneous" activity which renders the eliciting of reflexes difficult of evaluation. As a rule, it is almost impossible to determine whether a movement following stimulation was caused thereby or would have occurred without it.

By 25 weeks, all previous reflexes have greatly matured and the muscular system is increasing in strength. Self-sustained respiration, once begun, may last for over 24 hours. Tendon reflexes have become stronger and more complete. The eyelids may be opened and closed without stimulation by the observer and conjugate movements of the eyes, especially in the lateral plane, are evident. At this age, also, a Moro reflex was observed quite inadvertently. It may, therefore, be elicitable earlier. One fetus, lifted gently from the premature bed, in which it was being photographed, in order to change the underlying sheet which had been discolored by urination, was quickly lowered again. The almost clonic extension of arms and legs which resulted were typical of this "startle" reflex, which appears to have a vestibular origin.

Some obstetricians are of the opinion that a few 25-week premature infants may be viable. This is conceivably possible, although the youngest viable fetus observed in this series was 27 weeks of menstrual age. As previously noted (p. 62) all ages assigned in this study are menstrual ages. If by 25 weeks the so-called "corrected actual" age is intended, it would agree with 27 weeks of menstrual age. If 25 weeks of menstrual age is intended—and too often the exact kind of age used is not specified—it might still be possible, but not too probable in the light of the Pittsburgh observations. Possible viability at 27 weeks of menstrual age seems to agree with the majority opinion of obstetricians.

The 27-week fetus has greatly matured. The grasp of one was sufficiently strong to maintain with one hand practically its entire weight for a short period. In all examined at this or later ages the grasp is effective and the thumb participates most of the time, though feebly.

Little in the way of new responses appears from 27 weeks to birth, either at the usual 40 weeks or in such postmatures as have been observed. The suctorial response becomes matured into an active and audible sucking by 29 weeks. A definite cremasteric reflex has been observed by 32 weeks. At 33 weeks, the tongue may "search" the lower lip when that organ is lightly touched. For more details of the activities of the circumnatal period the reader is referred to the work of Arnold Gesell (1945). The number of fetuses observed in the Pittsburgh studies in this age range has been inadequate for final conclusions.

* * * * * *

Let us now turn our attention to a summary and discussion of the appearance and maturation of specific activities. First, however, it seems wise to review the spread of skin sensitivity to tactile stimulation.

At 7½ weeks, the sensitive area of the skin is closely limited to the area about the lips and alae of the nose, but by 8 through 9½ weeks the perioral region of sensitivity has widened slightly to include the chin and lateral parts about the mouth and nose. The facial area of sensitivity increases upward by 10½ weeks to include the eyelids in some and this region has become sensitive in most by 11 weeks. Two or three days after this (11½ weeks) the entire face is sensitive in all fetuses.

These are the areas supplied by the trigeminal nerve. In man it has been impossible to distinguish with certainty whether the skin area supplied by the maxillary or the mandibular divisions (V_2 or V_3) of this nerve becomes sensitive first. As already noted, Barcroft and Barron (1939a) stated that in the sheep the skin area supplied by V_2 becomes sensitive first. Indeed, in the sheep, V_3 does not mediate widespread responses, but V_1 does. In the Pittsburgh studies it was thought earlier that the V_2 area might precede the V_3 in becoming sensitive to stimulation in human embryos, but later cases have indicated that such an assumption is unwarranted. The area on the sides of the face toward the ears does not become sensitive much before 14 to 15 weeks, and the back and top of the head apparently remain insensitive until birth.

The palms of the hands become sensitive to tactile stimulation in a few cases early in the 10th week, apparently very slightly preceding the appearance of sensitivity in the skin of the arms and forearms, and of that in the soles of the feet, also found in a few specimens only. By 11 weeks all fetuses observed exhibited responses to palmar stimulation and most to stimulation over the arms and forearms. Although only some showed evidence of sensitivity of the sole of the foot at this age, all did so by 12 weeks. Sensitivity of the skin of the thighs and legs appeared slightly later than on the soles of the feet.

In response to appropriate stimulation, the first movement executed by the embryo is a contralateral flexion of the neck at about 7½ weeks. By about 8 weeks the upper trunk is included in the usually contralateral flexion and the upper extremities quiver as if attempting to participate, but are not otherwise involved in the response. From shortly after 8 weeks to 8½ weeks the typical response is a contralateral flexion of the neck and an increasingly caudalward-extending portion of the trunk, accompanied by extension of both arms at the shoulder, and some pelvic rotation. Between 8½ and 9½ weeks, the contralateral flexion of the trunk extends still farther caudally, and the hips exhibit a progressively more marked rotation toward the side of the trunk flexion. The arm extension at the shoulder does not alter its character in this period.

The caudally expanding response just outlined is evoked by unilateral stimulation with a 10 mg. or heavier hair stroked in the perioral region supplied by the maxillary and mandibular divisions of V. It may also be evoked at 9½ weeks by rotation of the embryo. From 7½ to at least 10 weeks of age, this is the only skin area of the body sensitive to such light stimulation. The use of heavy (stiff) hairs may cause local contractions of the longitudinal trunk muscles due to direct mechanical stimulation of the muscle tissue. Proprioceptive responses of the bineuronal stretch type may be elicited from forearm or brachial muscles by 9½ weeks. Evidence is lacking in these studies as to whether stretch reflexes may be elicited earlier, but Fitzgerald and Windle (1942) report responses of this type at 7½ weeks. The response given to unilateral perioral stimulation with a light hair is patterned and stereotyped. It is typically contralateral, but may more rarely be ipsilateral.

By 10½ weeks, trunk extension begins to replace the usual contralateral trunk flexion and by 11 to 12 weeks, extension has become the primary type of response to unilateral stimulation in the perioral area. This type of activity is usually accompanied by more or less marked medial rotation of the brachia. Neck rotation, turning the face away from the source of stimulation, occurs occasionally by 11 weeks and becomes more evident by 12 weeks and thereafter. By 13½ to 14 weeks, the trunk movements generally cease to be patterned and local activities of many kinds replace the larger responses.

Contractions limited to the chest make their appearance in the 18th week. This is possibly the age at which true respiratory movements first appear in human fetuses in good condition. Gasping, with agonal chest contractions, has been seen as early as 13 weeks in dying fetuses, but they have never been seen in cases of that early age when oxygen was being supplied to the placenta. However, Windle, Dragstedt, Murray, and Greene (1938) report respiratory movements of the chest in a fetus of 62 mm. CR (12 weeks). Chest contractions in the 18th week are not agonal in character and occur whether or not oxygen is being supplied to the placenta. These contractions are slight and occur over the more caudal half of the thorax. They may be elicited by gently stroking the chest with a 2 gm. hair.

By 20 weeks, these contractions have increased in amplitude and at 22 weeks are accompanied by expansions and contractions of the abdomen. Such abdominal expansions are unquestionably caused by activity of the diaphragm, the contractions of which compress the abdominal contents caudalward, as in adult respiration. Such activity, even at 22 weeks, is ineffectual. It has not been possible to resuscitate a fetus, even temporarily, before 23½ weeks, although examination of a greater number of cases might have shown earlier incidence of self-sustained respiration.

The time of beginning effective respiration appears to be dependent upon the level of development of the lungs, especially of its elastic tissue, which becomes differentiated at about 28 weeks (Hewer, 1938). When abdominal movements begin, the volume of the chest cavity is little, if at all, increased. When the diaphragm contracts, the lower thorax is drawn inward to create a relatively deep transverse depression over the lower rib-cage, deepest in the region of the xiphoid cartilage. This drawing inward of the lower ventral thoracic wall appears to compensate for the increase in vertical diameter of the thoracic cavity caused by the diaphragmatic contraction. At the time when sustained respiration becomes possible, the depth of the depression begins to diminish and, although it persists in some fetuses for many weeks, continues to become less evident. The last evidence of the depression lies over the xiphoid cartilage.

Originally regarded as a sign inimical to a good prognosis for survival, it has since been proved that older premature infants exhibiting some depression may nonetheless continue to live and thrive. Belief that the depression of the chest is caused by inadequate development of the lungs so that they are as yet incapable of filling the expanded thoracic cavity is based largely on assumption, but is strengthened by attempts to inflate the fresh lung. Though inadequate to prove the point, these inflation attempts indicate a relatively rapid increase in lung volume between 18 and 25 weeks. The gradual disappearance of the ventral depression during this period of growth further increases the possibility that the level of lung growth is largely responsible for viability of the premature infant.

At 23½ weeks, respiration, self-sustained for 2½ hours after resuscitation, was first accomplished. As attempts at resuscitation were carried to older ages, it was found that the duration of self-sustained respiration increased with age, as might be expected. At 24½ weeks, the duration of such respiration was 4½ hours; at 25 weeks, 26½ hours; and at 27 weeks, one premature continued to live.

Although the facial area is the only region sensitive to light tactile stimulation during the early reactions of the embryo, the facial muscles do not participate in responses of other components of the body and do not themselves exhibit movements before 10 to 10½ weeks. At that age contraction of the orbicularis oculi muscle may occasionally be elicited in response to stimulation of the upper lid. By 11 weeks, the corrugator muscle often participates in the response of the orbicularis, causing scowling as well as "squinting" of the eyelids. These occasional responses become quite constant between 12 and 13 weeks of age when an upper eyelid is stimulated. Eyelid "squinting" has once been observed following lower lip stimulation at 13 weeks and upper lip stimulation at 14 weeks. At 13 to 14 weeks, unilateral stimulation near the nose or upper lip causes an ipsilateral contraction of the quadratus labii superioris muscle, producing a sneering expression.

The eyes themselves are difficult to observe before the lids separate. However, what appeared to be conjugate depression of both eyes was observed through the closed lids in two fetuses of 12½ weeks of age. Beginning at 25 weeks conjugate lateral movements of the eyes have been seen when the lids were open, and at older ages conjugate eye movements in all directions have been observed.

Momentary lip closure may be elicited as early as 12½ weeks when the rima oris is touched and repetition of such stimulation may evoke swallowing at this age. Within 2 weeks deglutition becomes an almost constant finding on repeated lip stimulation. By 13 weeks, light touch on either lip causes its firm closure, maintained for an appreciable period of time. Upper lip stimulation at the rima oris evokes its protrusion at about 17 weeks, but a similar response of the lower lip has not been exhibited before 20 weeks. At 22 weeks, simultaneous protrusion of both lips results in pursing of the mouth. Definite, indeed audible, suction has been observed at 29 weeks, but may occur earlier.

The upper extremities slightly precede the lower in participation in trunk responses and in exhibiting specific reflexes. Just after 8 weeks, both brachia extend at the shoulder as part of the trunk response to unilateral stimulation about the mouth. The quivering of the upper extremity, including the fingers, observed in one case just before 8 weeks is almost certainly preliminary to the shoulder extension. At 10½ weeks, independent extension of one arm at the shoulder has been observed on stimulation of the shoulder. This response is rare, however, and occurred in a fetus in which partial finger closure had been elicited. Partial finger closure on light palmar stimulation is a constant response by 11 weeks, but may occur occasionally 3 to 5 days earlier. In these early cases of finger closure on palmar stimulation, medial rotation of the brachia, flexion of the elbow and forearm pronation have also been observed, but these likewise are rare findings. By 11½ weeks, medial rotation of the arms at the shoulder is a constant finding on perioral stimulation. Abduction of the arm at the shoulder in response to lateral brachial stimulation has been observed once at this age.

Coghill noted in *Amblystoma*, as has Youngstrom (1938) in *Rana, Bufo, Acris*, and other anurans, that specific limb responses appear in a proximodistal direction. Angulo (1932*b*) has noted that the same principle holds for the rat. Barron (1950) has called attention to the earlier ontogenetic development of both structure and function in the limbs of mammals in contrast to those of amphibians. This fact appears correlated with the earlier importance of the limbs in the former class of animals. Insofar as the Pittsburgh studies afford evidence, the human fetus appears to be further modified than the rat and other similar mammals in that, as noted, the strict proximodistal appearance of limb reflexes is only partially true. It may be that a greater number of sensory endings per unit area in the hand of man has led to the earlier development of its reflexes.

Halverson (1937, 1943) has made a careful study of prehension in infants and very young children. He notes that there are two successive steps in its development. The first of these is finger closure, the second, grasp. It is significant that in fetal life the same two steps are evident in the appearance of reflexes of the fingers (Hooker, 1938). In this and many other activities, postnatally developed voluntary acts appear in the same sequence in which they are elicitable as reflexes during fetal life. Attention might be called here to the unquestioned fact that the order of postnatal appearance of function on a voluntary basis must mirror the order of appearance of the antecedent fetal reflexes.

Finger closure, only partial and usually without the participation of the pollex, first appears between 10½ and 11 weeks on stimulation of the palm. It is soon accompanied by wrist flexion. Closure of the fingers becomes complete between 13½ and 14 weeks, at about which time thumb opposition has been observed. By 14 weeks there is a tendency for finger closure to be maintained for a brief period, but anything resembling true grasp does not appear for another week and becomes effective only by about 18½ weeks. By 27 weeks, however, the grasp may be sufficiently strong to support almost the entire weight of the body with one hand. It has proved practically impossible to induce a fetus to grasp with both hands at the same time until the circumnatal period.

In the lower extremity, aside from the rump rotation which, like the arm extension at the shoulder, is part of the trunk response, the toes respond to stimulation of the sole a little before responses of the thighs and legs may be elicited. Occasionally, plantar flexion of the toes may be elicited in more advanced fetuses a little over 10½ weeks of age. By 11½ weeks, the toes constantly respond to sole stimulation. The response may be either plantar flexion or dorsiflexion. Some fetuses appear to exhibit one or the other with greater facility, but almost all show both types of response on successive stimulation. At 11½ weeks, toe responses may be accompanied by flexion of the knee and at first flexion, then extension at the hip, resulting in a kick. Within a week (12 to 12½ weeks) and thereafter, response to sole stimulation consists principally of dorsiflexion of the hallux, with toe fanning, dorsiflexion of the foot at the ankle, and flexion at knee and hip.

* * * * * *

These, then, are the principal results of the Pittsburgh studies on the physiological responses of human embryos and fetuses. There is much yet to be done. Many aspects of reactive behavior have not even been attempted as yet, e.g., no studies on the functioning of the organs of special sense have been made. In other regards, only an inconclusive beginning has been made. It is hoped that progress will be made along these lines as the studies are continued.

Chapter 3

The Significance of Structural and Functional Interrelationships in Prenatal Activity

In the two preceding chapters, the more significant contributions on vertebrate embryonic and fetal overt behavior have been reviewed and the current results of an intensive study of human fetal activity have been presented. The review has indicated that various investigators, even in studies on one vertebrate class, have secured widely varying data. This is perhaps to be expected, as so many variables exist, and too many students of this complex problem have fastened their attention upon this or that aspect to the exclusion of others. Before the whole question of the development of activity throughout the vertebrate series will be solved, additional carefully planned and controlled observations must be made.

In the foregoing accounts, attention has been given to overt behavior alone. Very nearly the only indication that this externally visible activity is dependent upon the internal organization of the developing embryo, larva, or fetus has been the often repeated mention of the neuromuscular mechanism of the organism. Any living thing exists in an external environment. However, every living thing has an internal organization, which in most invertebrates and all vertebrates takes the form of organ systems. The interaction of the activities of these organ systems upon one another constitutes the internal environment of the whole animal. Furthermore, each organ system exists in an environment composed in part of elements of the external environment of the whole creature and in part of the elements furnished by the activities of other interacting organ systems. This is especially true of an adult vertebrate, but it is also true of one which is developing. The chief difference is that, in the developing organism, no organ system can act upon another until it has itself begun to function.

It is now proposed to explore the nature of the functional interactions of those mammalian organ systems which are important in development and such structural elements, especially of the nervous system, as have significance. The elements of the neuromuscular mechanism, which appear to be the sole source of the initial activity of the embryo, will be considered first. Not only are they of supreme importance for an understanding of embryonic activity, but there is perhaps more known about them than concerning almost any other component of the younger embryos.

The morphological development to functional capacity of the muscles, one of the two components of the neuromuscular mechanism of the embryo, is fairly well understood. The mesenchymal cells, from which the muscles arise, develop into mononucleated spindle-shaped myoblasts. As these elongate, their originally rather homogeneous cytoplasm exhibits longitudinal striations, the myofibrillae, which are at first clear (Straus and Weddell, 1940, in the rat), shortly become beaded, and finally are transformed into the definitive striated fibrils of skeletal muscle. The myofibrillae tend to be very few in number at first and to be located peripherally. Toward the center of the fiber the relatively large nuclei increase in number, probably by their amitotic division (LeGros Clark, 1945).

Whether or not myofibrillae are an essential component of mammalian skeletal muscle cells before they may exhibit contractility is not yet determined. The work of Goss (1940) indicates that cardiac muscle in the rat embryo begins its contractions while in a completely undifferentiated state. However, the fact remains that skeletal muscle fibers, when they first become functional, possess myofibrillae, although in very small numbers (Straus and Weddell, 1940, and unpublished observations on the Pittsburgh material).

As noted in the first chapter (p. 6), muscle activity may be classified as myogenic, neurogenic, or reflexogenic. It is certain that no spontaneous myogenic activity occurs in mammalian skeletal muscle. Whether such muscle may be mechanically or electrically excited to contraction without the intervention of motor nerves is as yet an incompletely settled problem. Straus and Weddell (1940) believe that all skeletal muscle in rat embryos, capable of being electrically excited to contraction, has a nerve supply and that the responses secured are not "myogenic" but neurogenic.

Neurogenic activity of skeletal muscle may be elicited only shortly before true reflexogenic action begins. As the skeletal muscle tissue in any vertebrate tends to differentiate in a progressively cephalocaudal direction, true reflexes may be elicited in the more cephalic (actually cervical) portions of an embryo before they can be secured from its more caudal elements.

The neural component of the neuromuscular mechanism develops within the central nervous system and the spinal ganglia. The motor neurons within the spinal cord precede the spinal ganglion cells in their differentiation. In all forms studied, motor fibers reach the primitive muscle-forming cell groups before differentiation in the latter has occurred. This is, of course, the reason why the neurogenic type of activity precedes, though by only a few hours, the reflexogenic.

Reflex activity requires, at a minimum, an afferent (sensory or receptor) and an efferent (motor or effector) neuron. Some proprioceptive reflex arcs are believed to be bineuronal, but exteroceptive arcs are considered to be multineuronal, having one or more association neurons intercalated between the receptor and the effector cells (Lloyd, 1943*a*, 1943*b*). It seems probable, though proof is lacking, that it is the synaptic connections which are the last elements of the arc to become functional in development and, thus, establish the integrity of the reflex arc.

It seems doubtful that the spinal ganglion cells begin to function as early as the cells of the semilunar (Gasserian) ganglion, as Windle (1934*a*, 1934*b*) believes they do. Angulo (1951*a*, 1951*b*) has shown that rat embryos of 264 hours fertilization age exhibit advanced fibrillation in the trigeminal ganglion, but that no neurofibrillae are present in the cervical ganglia before 288 hours. Responses to exteroceptive stimulation in the rat do not appear before 378 hours, according to Angulo. Thus the semilunar ganglion cells are well in advance of the spinal ganglion cells in differentiation in the rat. Much the same condition appears to exist in the human embryo.

Some authorities (Ranson, 1943; Clark, 1947) have denied that mammalian embryos can exhibit a response pattern basically similar to that of *Amblystoma* because of the absence of intramedullary ganglion cells in the mammalian spinal cord. That intramedullary sensory ganglion cells are actually present in the human embryonic spinal cord has been amply shown both by Humphrey (1944) and Youngstrom (1944), independently. Humphrey demonstrated two generations of these primitive intramedullary sensory neurons, the second of which is more numerous at the beginning of activity than at any other time. As they are predominantly present in the more caudal portions of the cord, they can play no role in the initial neck, trunk, and upper limb responses. However, Humphrey has suggested (1952*a*) that they may well participate, perhaps with the spinal ganglia, in the return to posture of the pelvic region in slightly older embryos. There appears to be no other evidence of the functioning of the spinal ganglion cells in the earliest responses. Indeed, all available indications point to the trigeminal nerve as mediating these earliest exteroceptive reflexes.

The work of a considerable number of investigators substantiates the view that external stimuli are first perceived in the facial region. Some term it the snout, some the perioral region, but all of these are merely brief ways of denoting that region of the face supplied by the trigeminal nerve.

The trigeminal nerve terminations are probably the earliest sensory receptors of the body (Windle, 1933; Angulo, 1936). The problem has been to trace the reflex pathway from V to the final common path in the spinal cord. The difficulty here has been to determine, morphologically, the caudal extent in the spinal tract of V of each of its divisions through the medulla and into the spinal cord. The fifth cranial nerve rarely stains or infiltrates with silver in a differential manner, contrasting it with other neighboring structures. Furthermore, animal operative experimentation and clinical postoperative observations have led to contradictory results.

It has been generally accepted, as a result of functional losses from accidental or operative injuries to the spinal tract of V, that mandibular division (V_3) fibers leave the tract to enter its spinal nucleus in its most cephalic part, that maxillary division (V_2) fibers leave next and that ophthalmic division (V_1) fibers alone extend to the caudal limits of the tract. Among those whose work led to this concept are Bregmann (1892) and Wallenberg (1896), who carried out experimental tract sections on rabbits, and a considerable group of clinicians who largely studied accidental "natural experiments" injuring the tract, including Schlesinger (1895), von Sölder (1899), Kutner and Kramer (1907), Spiller (1908), van Valkenburg (1911), Winkler (1921), Stopford (1924), Sjöqvist (1938), and Smyth (1939).

The exact point of termination of the fibers of V_2 and V_3 varies somewhat as given by different individuals. However, the majority opinion is that the fibers of these two divisions leave the descending root of V above the beginning of the spinal cord. Bregmann, van Valkenburg, Winkler, and Sjöqvist have stood almost alone in believing that V_2 and V_3 may extend to or into the first cervical segment (C1) of the spinal cord. Actually, van Valkenburg presents material that can be interpreted to indicate that some V_2 and V_3 fibers may pass as far caudally in the descending tract as C3 in man, though he does not so state in his descriptions.

There is some evidence suggesting that the representation of each division may vary according to the animal form. Barcroft and Barron (1939a) doubt that the fibers of V_3 in the sheep contribute any component to the descending tract of V on the basis of their finding that this division does not participate in the early trunk reflexes. They propose a pathway for the earliest reflexes of the sheep, which are otherwise quite similar to those described in the Pittsburgh studies for man, as follows: fibers of V2 through the semilunar ganglion into the descending spinal tract of V, thence into the reticular formation to establish contact with the cells of origin of the reticulo-spinal tract which, in turn, synapses with the lower motor neurons at varying levels of the spinal cord. This is not only an entirely possible reflex pathway from face to cervical cord, but one for which there is considerable morphological evidence. Furthermore, it does not require any further caudalward extension of V_2 in the spinal tract than that provided by the work of previous investigators.

Recently, the morphological studies of Humphrey (1951, 1952a) have provided an alternate and more probable pathway for the earliest reflexes elicited by perioral stimulation. In a detailed survey of the Pittsburgh collection of sectioned tested human embryos, three of them showed a differential silver impregnation which makes the spinal tract of V clearly identifiable, marking it off from the other longitudinal tracts of the dorsolateral quadrants of the medulla and spinal cord.

The fibers of the three divisions of V have a well-known arrangement (Bregmann, 1892, and others) in the spinal tract of V, the fibers of V_3 being most dorsal, those of V_2 in the middle and of V_1 ventral. Thus, Humphrey found it possible to determine the general position of the fibers of each of the divisions of V, even though they were not differentially colored by the silver. Furthermore, there is a persistence in adult man of the lateral notch in the spinal root of V which marks the phylogenetically ancient fusion of the originally separate ophthalmic nerve with the maxillomandibular fibers. Thus, although it is only possible to distinguish the general fiber area belonging to V_2 from that of V_3, the maxillomandibular complex can readily be distinguished from the fiber mass of V_1.

Because the arrangement of the ophthalmic and maxillomandibular fiber groups in the spinal tract of V is obviously the same in the human embryo as has been demonstrated for the adult, it was possible for Humphrey to plot the area occupied by V_1 and by V_2-V_3 in the spinal tract of V throughout its length and to establish their caudal limits in each of the three embryos which showed differential silver impregnation of the trigeminal fibers. These three were: 22 mm. CR (8— weeks), 25 mm. CR (8— weeks) and 26.5 mm. CR (8.5— weeks), the age period during which responses first appear on stimulation of the maxillomandibular distribution of V to the face.

Humphrey's findings[7] may be summarized as follows: 1) in the 22 mm. CR embryo, V_1 fibers end in the upper part to the middle of C2, but the fibers of the V_2-V_3 complex may be traced to C3; 2) in the 25 mm. CR embryo, V_1 fibers again end in mid-C2, the V_2-V_3 fibers extending to lower C2 or upper C3; 3) in the 26.5 mm. CR embryo, V_1 fibers still end in mid-C2, but the V_2-V_3 fibers extend to or into C4. The caudal extent of each fiber group differs slightly on the right and left sides of the embryo (fig. 5) and it must be borne in mind that, even though V_1 remains near mid-C2 throughout this age period, its fibers have

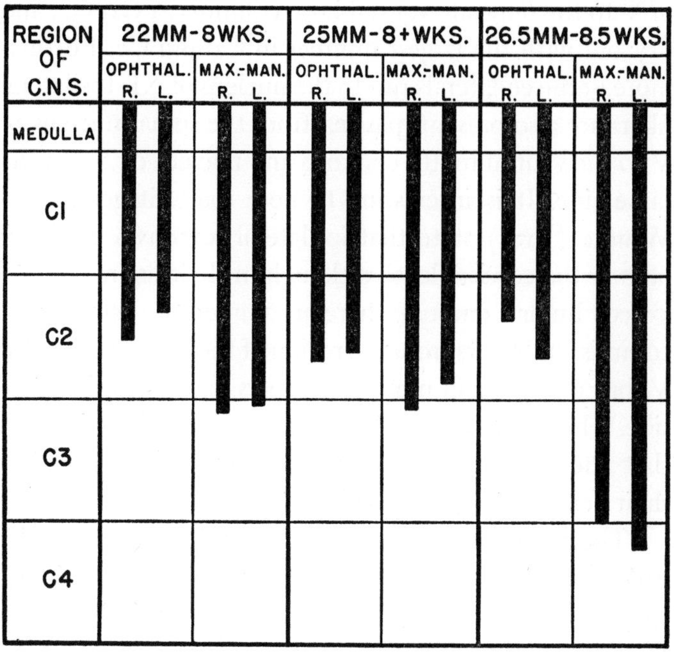

REGION OF C.N.S.	22MM-8WKS.				25MM-8+WKS.				26.5MM-8.5WKS.			
	OPHTHAL.		MAX.-MAN.		OPHTHAL.		MAX.-MAN.		OPHTHAL.		MAX.-MAN.	
	R.	L.	R.	L.	R.	L.	R.	L.	R.	L.	R.	L.
MEDULLA												
C1												
C2												
C3												
C4												

FIG. 5. Diagram of the caudal extent of the ophthalmic and maxillomandibular fibers in the spinal tract of the trigeminal nerve in young human embryos. (Courtesy of Dr. Tryphena Humphrey.)

grown in length to keep pace with the increase in length of the embryo as a whole.

Thus, at the age when the maxillomandibular fibers of the trigeminal nerve are functioning as the sensory limb of the reflex arc for contralateral flexion on stimulation of the perioral area, these divisions are already well into the spinal cord. Indeed, they already extend farther caudally than has ever before been demonstrated satisfactorily. However, are there any connections between V_2 and V_3 and the ventral horn motor cells? Humphrey finds a wealth of commissural fibers from the region of the spinal nucleus of V to the opposite ventral horn columns in C1, C2, and C3, but with the largest number in C1 and C2. Furthermore, some collaterals run to the nucleus of XI. Ipsilateral fibers are also present, passing from the spinal nucleus of V to the ventral motor columns and nucleus of XI on the same side. It is interesting to note that Fitzgerald and Windle (1937) state that ipsilateral responses predominate in the cervical level, although in their figure 10, of a 5-week human embryo, there are numerous contralateral commissural fibers from the region of the spinal nucleus of V, but only a small number of fibers passing to the same side. This figure of Fitzgerald and Windle demonstrates that the commissural connections of V long antedate their being called into active function.

The reflex pathway presented by Humphrey for the earliest contralateral reflexes in human embryos in response to stimulation in the perioral region is as follows (fig. 6): 1) via the maxillomandibular divisions of V, through the semilunar ganglion and the spinal tract, to the spinal nucleus of V in the cervical cord; 2) thence predominantly by commissural fibers to the ventral motor cell columns of the opposite side, but with occasional ipsilateral discharges to these columns, and slightly later to the nuclei of XI on both sides; 3) then by cervical lower motor neurons to the neck and upper trunk muscles to produce the chiefly contralateral flexion in this region and by the neurons of XI on both sides to facilitate the bilateral extension of the arms at the shoulders.

Inasmuch as the maxillomandibular fibers of V are present in the cervical spinal cord and the commissural connections exist at the time when contralateral cervical flexion begins, movements during the early age period probably are mediated over this path. During later stages, however, it seems likely that the reticulo-spinal pathway suggested by Barcroft and Barron reinforces the response and increases its caudal extent in the cervical and thoracic regions of the spinal cord.

It would thus appear that there is a very definite reflex pathway which indicates that the activities observed in early human embryos and described in the preceding chapter (pp. 62-68) are true exteroceptive reflexes mediated over a morphologically demonstrated pathway. These exteroceptive reflexes are basic to both pre- and postnatal activities.

It now becomes necessary to examine the type or types of reflexes exhibited by the embryo in its initial responses and the pathways mediating them. Windle (1934*b*, 1944) and Windle and Fitzgerald (1937) believe that the initial reflex arcs to become functional in cat and human embryos lie exclusively in the cervical cord, reaching its peak of development in the brachial plexus region. It will be recalled (pp. 36, 47) that Swenson (1929) and Windle (1936) and his co-workers are of the opinion that behavior in the mammal has its origin "in simple, non-integrated, spinal type reflexes" (Windle, p. 33*P*). Windle (1944 and elsewhere) has stated that the earliest limb reflexes elicited by him in various mammals by tapping the amnion or "flipping" a limb are proprioceptive reflexes but that the head reflex in response to amnion tapping is exteroceptive. If the limb flip response is a reflex, it is unquestionably of the stretch type and it might be maintained that the head reflex on amnion tapping could, at least sometimes, be of that type also. Any change in head-body relationships, even of an infinitesimal amount, may stretch the neck muscles and

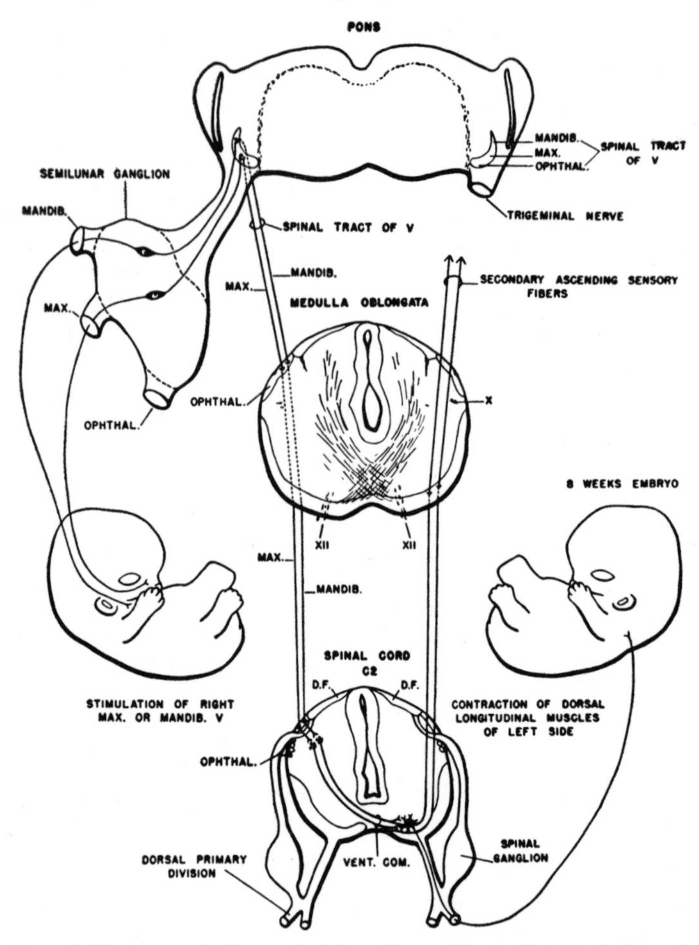

Fig. 6. Diagram of the probable reflex pathway for contralateral neck and upper trunk reflexes in the early human embryo. (From Humphrey, 1952a, by permission of the Wistar Institute of Anatomy and Biology.)

cause a proprioceptive reflex of this kind. All stretch reflexes are narrowly localized, and Windle's head responses from amnion tapping are as localized as his limb reflexes from the same kind of stimulation. Only those head responses secured by Windle and others in response to stimulation in the snout region can, with assurance, be termed exteroceptive. However, in the sheep, at least, there may be doubt that the limb flip response is a reflex. Barron (1944) has shown that reflex arcs are immature, if not incomplete, in this form when such motility is exhibited.

There has been much misunderstanding of Sherrington's (1906) term "the simple reflex." Even Coghill (1909) leaned somewhat toward the simple reflex as an entity, at first, but soon abandoned it as contrary to his findings. Because of the misunderstanding, it seems well to quote Sherrington's exact words (pp. 7-8):

> The simple reflex. There is the co-ordination which a reflex action introduces when it makes an effector organ responsive to excitement of a receptor, all other parts of the organism being supposed indifferent to or indifferent for that reaction. In this grade of co-ordination the reflex is taken apart, as if separable from all other reflex actions. This is the *simple reflex*. A simple reflex is probably a purely abstract conception, because all parts of the nervous system are connected together and no part of it is probably ever capable of reaction without affecting and being affected by various other parts, and it is a system certainly never at rest. But the simple reflex is a convenient, if not a probable, fiction. Reflexes are of various degrees of complexity, and it is helpful in analyzing complex reflexes to separate from them reflex components which we may consider apart and therefore treat as though they were simple reflexes.

Sherrington's discussion of the simple reflex clearly indicates its mythical character. Even in the adult, the most localized reflexes, of the stretch type, can occur only through the co-ordinated action of other nervous mechanisms, such as those which inhibit the response of antagonistic muscles. This is equally true of the embryo, despite the less complicated state of the nervous system in comparison with that in the adult.

According to the Windle concept, proprioceptive reflexes are not only early, they are the first to appear. However, the Pittsburgh studies have shown that definitely exteroceptive reflexes also appear in man at the age in which Fitzgerald and Windle (1942) first found proprioceptive reflexes. Thus it would appear that proprioceptive reflexes do not precede those of exteroceptive nature in being manifested, although they may appear almost simultaneously.

Such an early appearance of proprioceptive reflexes may be indicative of their increasing importance in higher vertebrates, but there is no evidence that behavior patterns are built up from proprioceptive reflexes. On the contrary, all available evidence indicates that overt behavior is primarily the response of the organism as a whole to its external environment. This response is based on exteroceptive sense, with proprioceptive or interoceptive reactions as incidental modifying factors. Thus, even if the Swenson-Windle concept of unitary reflexes were to be accepted, it is very doubtful, especially if they are proprioceptive in nature, that they ever form the basis for the elaboration of behavior since they involve only a part of the organism.

Windle, Becker, Rhines, and Cowgill (1942) and Windle (1944, 1950*b*) have challenged the normal nature of all contralateral reflexes by the statement that responses are normally ipsilateral and become contralateral only as a result of asphyxia. This statement does not coincide with the findings of the Pittsburgh studies or with those of Angulo (1932*b*). Responses to stimulation in the perioral (or snout) region are very definitely contralateral in the vast majority of cases and are of this character from the beginning. Ipsilateral responses may occur following perioral stimulation, but they are relatively infrequent in both rat and man. Stimulation outside the perioral region in early reactive ages always produces ipsilateral responses. These are definitely caused by mechanical stimulation of the muscle tissue directly. There is no known mechanism for the reversal of this type of response into a contralateral form.

This statement by Windle leads directly to a consideration of the oxidation of tissues and related matters. After about the third week of fertilization age and the fifth of menstrual age, the embryo has a blood circulation, for the heart begins its beat at approximately that time. Prior to the initiation of the heart beat, some other mechanism must care for the oxygen needs of the dividing egg and the developing early embryo, as oxygen diffusion alone is inadequate. This mechanism appears to be found in the activities of the so-called oxidation-reduction enzymes. These enzymes are known to be widely present, particularly in early developing tissues, but are also active in later life. Indeed, although they appear to decrease in activity as development proceeds, little is known of the time at which they cease to have an effect, if such cessation ever occurs. All animal experiments have revealed a quite universal applicability of the chemical principles governing oxidation-reduction enzymes.

These enzymes facilitate three types of chemical reactions within the organism: "preparation" or conversion reactions, those concerned with dehydrogenation, and those aiding decarboxylation. Conversion reactions enter into the alteration of 2-carbon compounds, from which hydrogen cannot be separated, into 6-carbon compounds from which hydrogen may be lost. These reactions prepare embryonic compounds, especially for dehydrogenation, and alter the chemicals of food materials at almost all ages.

Dehydrogenation reactions assist in the liberation of hydrogen ions which are absorbed by the pyridine nucleotides, but their end result is to effect oxidation and to provide water. Decarboxylation reactions tend to liberate CO_2. In their activities, oxidation-reduction enzymes play an important role in glycolysis, which is an essential feature of nervous system respiration. Too little is known of the effectiveness of these enzymes once a circulation has been established. However, Ball (1952) has shown that they do act for adult nervous and other tissues under anoxial conditions.

Once a circulation is established, at about five weeks of menstrual age in the human embryo, it becomes one of the important elements in the internal environment of the embryo as a whole, as well as of the neuromuscular mechanism. The circulation is most important in any consideration of the activity of mammalian, and especially human, embryos. Here, more than in any other class of vertebrates, there is not only the danger, but the demonstrable fact, of greater or less interference with normal O_2-CO_2 interchanges in all of the tissues of the embryo. It is only because they are metabolically more active than other tissues or organ systems that nerve and muscle are particularly affected.

In the mammalian embryo and fetus, the O_2-CO_2 interchange, which occurs in the lungs of the postnatal individual, must take place in the placenta. Here the interchange of these gases between the embryo's own blood and the maternal blood takes place through the placental barriers interposed between the two blood streams. The maternal blood, in turn, is "aerated" in the mother's lungs.

The placental barriers, just mentioned, consist of the

layers of tissue separating the fetal from the maternal blood. The number of layers differs in different forms and the placentae of all mammals may be classified into five categories on the basis of the layers present (Grosser, 1927; Mossman, 1937). In spite of the differing number of layers of the placental barriers—from one to six, three in man—all placentae function on the same principle, although it appears that the thinner the barrier, the more efficient is the placenta (Barron, 1951).

As Barcroft (1947) points out, the oxygen demand of the fetal cells removes this gas from the fetal blood. This O_2 utilization lowers the oxygen pressure of the fetal blood below that of the maternal blood. In consequence, "there is thus a pressure gradient of oxygen foetus-wards" in the placenta (see also, Barron, 1946). Barcroft also calls attention to the fact that embryonic and fetal blood are quite different from the blood of the postnatal infant. Wintrobe and Shumacker (1936), working with the fetuses, prematures, and neonates of mammals, including man, have demonstrated that the red blood cells in early fetuses of all forms studied are unusually large in size, that most are nucleated, and that the hemoglobin per cell is high. At this time, the total number of red blood corpuscles and the total amount of hemoglobin are both relatively low. As development proceeds, the size of the red cells and the percentage of nucleated reds decrease, but the total amount of hemoglobin and the total number of red blood corpuscles increase. However, the hemoglobin per cell drops, so that the rise in total hemoglobin is not great. Barcroft (1947) calls attention to the general agreement among those who have studied fetal blood that the hemoglobin content, hence the oxygen capacity, of fetal blood rises during development, particularly in early embryos, younger than the smallest (51 mm. CR, about 11½ weeks) studied by Wintrobe and Shumacker. The initial rise in the amount of hemoglobin is rapid at first and then gradually slows to the relatively slight increment observed by Wintrobe and Shumacker. This means, of course, that the oxygen capacity of the early embryo is very low, in the sheep less than a third of that of the late fetus. In consequence, the amount of oxygen which embryonic blood is capable of carrying is low normally, at the time of beginning movements. Hence, the oxygen demand of embryos and young fetuses must be very small, far less than in older fetuses. This, also, is in agreement with the findings of many workers in this field, such as Windle (1950*a*), Barron (1950), and others.

The low oxygen capacity of the early embryo is evidently without untoward effect upon the activity of the primary reflex arcs. They have developed in a still lower oxygen environment and the greater supply at the time of their beginning function is entirely adequate. This is not the case, however, with newer neural mechanisms which become active later. It is particularly not the case in connection with those centers which have their synapses at higher levels of the central nervous system. There is a very definite gradient of oxygen demand in the central nervous system, which increases in the cephalic direction. Cannon and Burket (1913) gathered information determining the following survival times, under complete anoxial conditions, for the adult central nervous system: cerebrum, 8 minutes; cerebellum, 13 minutes; medulla, up to 30 minutes; and spinal cord, up to 60 minutes. This has been amply substantiated (Himwich, 1951, pp. 288-290). In addition all newer neural components which develop find a decreasing increment in oxygen supply, as mentioned in the last paragraph. Although growth is well taken care of in this respect, function is, at first, an added load not too well tolerated. As a result, there is a tendency for newer neural mechanisms at higher levels to succumb relatively early to the effects of anoxia and asphyxia. This causes a reversion in the behavior pattern to an earlier type of activity in young fetuses. The tendency to reversion has been found to be true for the rat by Angulo and has been noted in the Pittsburgh human fetal studies.

In primary reflexes, on the contrary, and particularly in those of exteroceptive type, quite other conditions prevail. Here the afferent fibers are of the smallest caliber. These are resistant to asphyxia, both in the experience of the Pittsburgh group and as indicated by Windle *et al.* (Windle and Becker, 1940; Fitzgerald and Windle, 1942; Windle, Becker, Rhines and Cowgill, 1942; Windle, 1950*b*) and by Houssay (1951). In view of the fact that the spinal cord has the lowest oxygen requirement of any region of the central nervous system, exteroceptive reflexes which are dependent on the cord for their synaptic transmission, as are those over the trigeminal nerve (fig. 6), should be the last to succumb to anoxia.

However, the effect of anoxia and asphyxia on reflexes is twofold. Not only are reflexes ultimately abolished by these conditions, but initially they are also facilitated by them. Sherrington (1910) was probably the first to note that a certain amount of asphyxia, in an adult cat, may facilitate the eliciting of reflexes. More recently, Brooks and Eccles (1947) have demonstrated that it is the anoxial component of asphyxia which produces hyperexcitability, as the excess of CO_2 has a purely depressant effect. This depression is, however, usually overridden, for a time, by the excitatory effect of the anoxia. That anoxia may facilitate reflexes in mammalian embryos has been noted by Angulo (1930*b*), Barron (1941), and Windle, Becker, Rhines, and Cowgill (1942). A more detailed analysis of the effects of anoxia on reflexes and on the development of early fetal activity is to be presented by Humphrey (1952*b*), and the reader is referred to her discussion for this and other aspects of the subject.

Windle *et al.* (1940, 1942) have reported an initial period, following immediately upon opening of the uterus, during which the cat embryo failed to respond to stimulation until the "brilliantly red" blood "began to darken" within a matter of seconds. Then responses to stimulation could be elicited and spontaneous activity soon appeared, particularly if the placenta of the cat fetus under examination was removed from the uterus. This initial period of no-response in the cat has been interpreted by these investigators as indicating that, under normal conditions in the intact animal, fetal movements do not occur and that early movements are only elicitable under the influence of the facilitatory action of anoxia.

However, it is by no means certain that early mammalian and human movements do not occur normally *in utero*. As far as man is concerned, it is a matter of common knowledge among obstetricians that, although the "quickening" is usually said to begin about the 16th to the 18th week of menstrual age, some patients "feel life" in the uterus as early as the 10th to the 14th week of a pregnancy for which the date of confinement is known to have been correctly estimated.

Actually, it is unimportant whether intra-uterine activity does occur normally *in utero* in the intact organism or not, as the nervous system continues to develop in either the normal or enforced absence of movements. Harrison (1904) placed frog embryos in a chloretone solution when swimming reflexes were first appearing and kept them anesthetized for 7 days. Seventeen minutes after being again placed in clear tap water, the embryos were capable of producing normal reactions for their age. Herrick and Coghill (1915), Coghill (1924*a*), and Matthews and Detwiler (1926) used chloretone solution on *Amblystoma* embryos with similar results. It is true that when embryos were kept for very long periods in a solution of chloretone, some interference with the metabolism of the organism resulted in slight retardation of development of portions of the nervous system, causing some atypical responses under these conditions. This is beside the point, as chloretone is a highly abnormal environment. These experiments clearly show that normal development may occur in the absence of motility and, indeed, Coghill (1924*b*) points out that the neuromuscular mechanisms for new types of reflexes, however complex, develop without functioning until "shunted" into the active system in a fully perfected state.

Concerning the initial no-response state reported by Windle and Becker (1940) and Windle, Becker, Rhines, and Cowgill (1942) for the cat, it must be borne in mind that infraprimate mammals may differ greatly from primates in the response of their embryos. Some years ago, a series of observations were made in Pittsburgh on rat fetuses placed under conditions identical with those obtaining for the Pittsburgh human embryonic and fetal observations. The rat embryos or fetuses were removed with the placenta, placed in warmed Tyrode's solution, and stimulated by hairs. The results indicate that the rat fetus does not act as does the human fetus of comparable developmental stages. Immediately following delivery, the rat fetus exhibits under these conditions a very brief period, limited to less than a minute, during which only strong stimulation, interpreted as direct mechanical stimulation of the muscle tissue, can evoke any movement. Such responses as are elicited are entirely local. This may correspond to Windle's period of no-response. Following this no-response period, there is another, extending over a few (2 to 3) minutes, during which reflexes of the exteroceptive type and corresponding to Angulo's (1932*b*) responses in rats of comparable age, may be secured. Reflexes then disappear, but spontaneous movements, which begin as soon as the reflexes, continue for periods of as long as ten minutes.

The human fetus acts quite differently. Spontaneous movements are not observed in all embryos, but those which exhibit them do so ordinarily only within the first minute after beginning placental separation. Embryos which are capable of reflexes and which exhibit spontaneous movements apparently lack a prolonged period of no-response. They react to external stimulation as soon as it is applied, between one and two minutes after beginning placental separation. Those embryos which do not exhibit spontaneous activity do have a very definite no-response period, lasting up to three minutes or more. This is followed by a period of response to external stimulation. By actual count, only 31 per cent of the embryos and fetuses, considered as unanesthetized and from 7½ through 14 weeks of age, exhibited a no-response period. These were believed to be the cases suffering somewhat more trauma during extraction than the 69 per cent which moved spontaneously and had no period during which reflexes could not be secured.

Exteroceptive responses may be evoked initially by hairs having 25 mg., or higher, pressure values. In a few instances, responses have been secured with 10 mg. hairs. After a few (2 to 3) minutes, a 50 mg. or stiffer, hair is necessary. In another minute or two, a 100 mg. hair is required. In other words, there is a steady rise in threshold until responses cease. In 7½- to 8½-week fetuses, this occurs within 5 to 8 minutes after beginning placental separation. Older fetuses respond over longer periods, up to 12 to 14 minutes at 14 weeks.

Whether Windle and Becker (1940) and Windle, Becker, Rhines, and Cowgill (1942) are correct in assigning the no-response period, when it occurs, to normal nonmotility or whether it is a phenomenon akin to surgical shock, either in whole or in part, is undetermined. Indeed, it does not greatly matter. Even if the earliest reflexes in the embryo should only appear when facilitated by anoxia, the character of such responses is unaffected by the anoxia (Kato, 1934; Brooks and Eccles, 1947; Humphrey, 1925*b*); hence the neuromuscular mechanism exhibits activity which is normal in character even under these conditions. Furthermore, anesthesia which does not obliterate a primary reflex entirely has little effect upon the nature of the reflex. If one includes all responsive human embryos and fetuses from 7½ through 14 weeks, instead of eliminating those under suspicion of anesthesia, it appears that 30 per cent showed a no-response period and 70 per cent exhibited none, but moved spontaneously and reacted as soon as tested. The fact that these figures correspond with those from the selected nonanesthetized group is an added bit of evidence confirming the contention of Kato (1934) and others that anesthesia, short of obliterating nerve conduction, has little effect upon the normal character of a response. Anesthesia may, however, delay the response or decrease the amplitude of the reaction as the anesthetic blocks transmission in some of the fibers within the nerve.

The Pittsburgh studies have thus demonstrated an unbroken series of continuously developing responses in man from 7½ weeks to the time when breathing can be established. These may be interpreted as indicating the normal sequence of neuromuscular potentialities for activity in human embryos and fetuses at the different ages. Except for the appearance of tendon reflexes after the establishment, even temporarily, of respiration, there are no qualitative differences in the responses of breathing and nonbreathing fetuses of the same age. All responses in the series are normal steps in the development of behavior, whether or not they are somewhat facilitated by anoxia, or whether or not the earliest occur *in utero*.

* * * * * *

The circulatory, muscular, and nervous systems of the mammalian embryo are the first to reach a morphological level which permits their beginning to function. In addition, the presence of oxidative-reductive enzymes aids tissue respiration. Regarding other organ systems, relatively little is definitely known, but that little should be noted, even though more or less in passing, if for no other reason than to indicate that their function may have significance. That any of these other organ systems affects early mammalian overt behavior, as such, appears very doubtful at this time, but their functioning forms a part of the internal environment of the organism, even though they may contribute little to covert behavior in the first half or more of gestation.

It has been generally assumed that, because the placenta carries out for the embryo and fetus the functions of lungs, urinary system, and the absorptive aspects of the digestive system, there is no need for these organs to begin function in the developing organism until shortly before or at the beginning of the viable period. Actually, these organs exhibit function of a sort as soon as they are capable of it.

The kidneys of the fetus begin to function at an early age. Guthmann and May (1930) proved the presence of urea and uric acid in small quantities in the amniotic fluid of a human fetus of about the tenth week. In the Pittsburgh studies, the bladder has sometimes been found to contain fluid at older ages (e.g., 15½, 20½, and 25 weeks). This fluid was proved to be a dilute urine in the 25-week specimen. In general, activity of fetuses causes emptying of the bladder, so that fluid is relatively seldom found at autopsy. Windle (1940) gives an excellent review of the literature on this subject. However, it appears hardly possible that kidney function can affect the fetus seriously, since the placenta can care for fetuses which lack kidneys, ureters, or bladder (Preyer, 1885, pp. 326 *et seq.*).

Alimentary canal function also occurs in mammalian fetuses. There is considerable doubt as to when various digestive juices are formed, but none regarding the facts of swallowing, peristalsis, and defecation. Preyer (1885) reviewed earlier studies. Becker, Windle, Barth, and Schulz (1940) have clearly demonstrated, by the injection of thorotrast into the amniotic fluid, that the guinea-pig fetus begins to swallow on about the 42nd day (gestation, 67-69 days), exhibits transport of the material through the alimentary canal, slowly at first, but with increasing speed as term is approached, and begins to defecate into the amniotic fluid about the 60th day. Yanase (1907) demonstrated peristalsis in mammalian and human fetuses. Although the Pittsburgh studies have demonstrated that the human fetus may swallow as early as 12½ weeks, it was not until 1946 that Davis and Potter demonstrated the presence of thorotrast, injected into the amniotic fluid, in the alimentary canal of human fetuses as early as 75 mm. in length (13 weeks). Windle and Bishop (1939) and Becker *et al.* (1940) are of the opinion that fetal anoxia tends to stimulate earlier deglutition, and Windle has criticized the results observed by Davis and Potter on the basis of fetal asphyxia. As yet, there is no evidence that the human fetus normally defecates *in utero*. Here, again, it seems unlikely that alimentary function seriously affects the overt activities of the fetus.

The question of normal mammalian intra-uterine respiration is still in dispute, despite the fact that discussion of this phenomenon began long ago. Preyer (1885), who added personal observations of his own, notes that Vesalius observed respiratory movements in fetuses of dog and pig, and that a not inconsiderable number of early eighteenth century observers of mammalian fetuses, including those of man, have recorded their data on respiration. In the early observations, speculation was rife, as Preyer points out, regarding the cause or causes of early mammalian respiration, whether it was anoxia and excess of CO_2, external stimulation, or both working together.

Ahlfeld and his associates, over a period of years (1888 to 1905), observed certain rhythmic activities of the human fetus *in utero* and in 1905 summarized the results obtained and the conclusions drawn. These fetal movements had a rate of 38 to 80 per minute at different ages, and were not synchronous with the material aortic beat or respiration, but were distinct from the abdominal movements of the mother. Ahlfeld therefore concluded that these fetal activities were respiratory movements. Although criticism of Ahlfeld's work was severe, others also reported somewhat similar results (e.g., Reifferscheid, 1911).

A considerable number of observers have reported finding lanugo, bits of vernix caseosa, and other detritus from the amniotic fluid in the respiratory passages of still-born infants or those which had died shortly after birth. Such findings are not clear-cut evidence of normal intra-uterine respiration, however, although they aid in demonstrating that the respiratory apparatus can function to some extent at very early ages.

Barcroft and Barron (1936) found that mere handling of the sheep fetuses could start rhythmic respiratory type movements between 38 and 49 days (gestation 157 days). Such movements could not be excited at this stage by asphyxial conditions of the blood. The rhythm continued for relatively long periods of time, when once begun, but disappeared after the 50th day unless the umbilical cord were clamped. In early stages, at least, there was no aspiration of amniotic fluid, as negative pressure was not established in the lungs.

Snyder, with Rosenfeld (1936, 1937*a*, 1937*b*, 1937*c*) inhibited parturition in the rabbit and found that fetuses between 28 and 34 days (gestation 32 days) exhibited spontaneous rhythmic respiratory activity. Such activity could be suppressed by injections of phenobarbital sodium into the fetus. They concluded that intra-uterine respiration of amniotic fluid during the latter part of pregnancy is a normal occurrence in the mammalian fetus, indeed, an essential step in the development of the lungs, as the hydrostatic effect of inspired amniotic fluid serves to mold the alveoli. In this latter opinion they are in agreement with Wislocki (1920) and Bremer (1935). Snyder and Rosenfeld (1937a) state that anoxia depresses and ultimately abolishes these rhythmic activities, but that CO_2 is necessary to maintain them, although the amount required is not critical.

Windle and his associates (1938 to 1950) have carried out a considerable number of observations and experiments on fetal respiration. Steele and Windle (1939) were earlier convinced that, in the cat, fetal breathing shortly before term might be a normal intra-uterine procedure, but Windle, Becker, Barth, and Schulz (1939) later determined in the guinea-pig fetus that fetal intra-uterine respiratory movements are executed only under asphyxial conditions and are not accompanied by aspiration of amniotic fluid in all cases.

Opposed to this is the work of Davis and Potter (1946), who observed inspiration of thorotrast-laden amniotic fluid into the lungs of human fetuses between 75 and 300 mm. CR, which were about to be removed from the uterus for well-substantiated medical reasons. As already noted, this work has been adversely criticized by Windle.

In view of the unreconciled evidence presented, more work in this field may be expected. About all that has been clearly proved is that the respiratory apparatus is capable of some degree of function at a very early fetal age in man and other mammals.

In spite of the enormous number of contributions in the literature, present-day knowledge regarding the time in fetal life at which each of the endocrine organs may become functional is still confused and incomplete. The situation is further complicated by the fact that at least some hormones of maternal origin unquestionably pass through the placenta from mother to fetus, and no criterion exists for the separation of these maternal hormones from those elaborated by the fetus itself. Efforts have been, and are being, directed toward gaining further information regarding the time at which fetal endocrine organs may begin to elaborate their own secretions, the fetal age at which each hormone becomes available in sufficient quantity to affect its target organ, and the stage in development at which the target organ may be affected by hormones of either fetal or maternal origin.

As yet, the methods used in securing such information have proved inadequate in most cases for an exact solution of the problems presented. Some of the means used are morphological, some have employed implantation of fetal organs in immature postnatal animals to test their potency, and some have used feeding tests or microchemical methods of analysis. Each has its pitfalls, but each provides some information which may throw light in the dark corners.

As neither space nor the purpose of this inquiry permits an exhaustive review of the information even now available, only a few references to the subject, illustrating our present knowledge in the field, will be given here. The interested reader may refer to the excellent reviews of Moore (1947, 1950) for a detailed account and the references to the literature.

The goal of the morphological studies has been to determine by histological examination, often with special stains or impregnations, when the cytological structure of endocrine cells reaches a level of development resembling that of adult cells known to produce secretion and thereby to estimate the fetal age at which these cells might secrete. Except insofar as such cytological examination meets the requirements of appropriate microchemical tests, there is no evidence available that the attainment of a given level of differentiation can be accepted as corresponding with the beginning of function. In muscle tissues, nervous tissues, and some other organs, the attempt to estimate functional level from cytological structure has proved deceptive and unreliable. Nevertheless, in the case of some endocrine organs, there has been a reasonably close agreement between the results of histological estimations and of tests for physiological activity. In others, there has been wide discrepancy.

In the pituitary gland, morphological studies indicate that the alpha cells of the pars distalis achieve the appearance of functional capacity at varying fetal ages in different forms. In man, this appearance is reached early, at about 12 weeks, but no tests for physiological activity have as yet been made. The same is true in marsupials, where the histologically estimated age of initial functional possibility is about 11 or 12 days, one or two days after the young reach the pouch. In both these forms, the cytological evidence indicates a very early possible beginning of secretion. However, in the pig and guinea pig, morphological evidence points to a midfetal date for the possible beginning of function and these animals are born in a more advanced condition of development than are marsupials and man. In the case of the pig, implantation or feeding tests of physiological activity of the fetal pituitary indicate that gonadotropic hormone is not present until a week or two after the midfetal period and thyrotropic hormone is not effective until shortly before birth. It must, of course, be borne in mind that the time of beginning secretion and the time of production of secretion in sufficient quantity to be effective on a postnatal target organ may well be widely separated from one another.

In the developing thyroid, colloid has been demonstrated in the Pittsburgh embryos at 10 weeks of menstrual age, but again tests for physiological activity are lacking. In the rat, thyroids from 17-day fetuses failed to metamorphose amphibian larvae, but those from 18-day fetuses did so, and radioactive iodine has been shown to be stored in the thyroids of 19-day fetuses.

The androgenic, or fetal, cortex or X-zone of the human suprarenal is very large beginning with the third fetal month, but begins involution at about normal term. Involution is not completed until toward the end of the neonatal period. However, no tests for physiological activity of the human suprarenal androgenic zone have been successful during either the fetal or neonatal period. It is interesting to note that the X-zone disappears from the suprarenal of prematurely born infants within about 30 days. In some cases the premature attains the postneonatal state a month or more before it would have done so had it remained *in utero* until normal term. The question naturally arises, therefore, whether the supply of maternal hormone passed to the fetus through the placenta maintains the adrenal androgenic zone until birth. Reports on adrenal medullary function in human and other mammalian fetuses are conflicting, and work on the generalized cortex has failed to produce evidence of secretion.

Studies of pancreatic islet function have established that insulin is present in the pancreas of the 5-month-old calf in somewhat greater proportional amounts than in the adult organ. Aside from this one demonstrated fact, puzzling contradictions appear. What appeared to be conclusive evidence that insulin secreted by dog fetuses might pass into the maternal blood and improve the condition of the depancreatized diabetic mother (Carlson and Drennan, 1911) received a rude shock from the work of Cuthbert *et al.* (1940), who substantiated the earlier work, but also showed similar maintenance of the bitch during nursing of the pups.

Histological studies have also proved confusing because of the differences found in various forms. Alpha cells are said not to be present before birth in the rat, the beta (insulin-secreting) cells existing alone. Yet Donaldson and Humphrey (1949) have shown that argentophilic cells (considered by Ferner, 1938, and Hultquist, 1946, to be alpha cells) are present in the human pancreas during the 9th week of menstrual age. Aggregates, containing both argentophilic and other cells, considered to be islet tissue (Humphrey and Donaldson, 1949) are present at 10 weeks.

The interstitial cells of the human testis are more prominent in the 14- or 15-week fetus than in the adult, but the exact stage at which they may begin secretion is still unknown. Study of the so-called freemartin has indicated, however, that their function probably begins early. Cattle twins almost invariably form connections between the two fetal membranes, with a continuity between the chorioallantoic blood vessels of each resulting. Where one twin is male and the other female, the latter's internal reproductive system exhibits abnormalities of development which fail to occur if both twins are females. The freemartin has female external genitalia, but the internal organs become largely those of the male sex. As testicular development in the male precedes the ovary in differentiation, it is believed that male secondary sex hormones secreted by the interstitial cells of the male twin effect the maintenance of the male organs of the female twin and the degeneration or atrophy of her female organs. A somewhat similar effect is sometimes seen in the pig, but has not received the careful study given the freemartin by Lillie (1917) and others. The results of the injection of androgens and estrogens into pregnant female animals has further confounded confusion. Androgens might be expected to produce freemartin-like changes in female offspring when so injected and do, with certain differences. However, estrogens, similarly injected, tended to produce results somewhat similar to those of androgens. To top this, the feeding experiments of Warkany showed that maternal low vitamin A diets tended to produce results similar to those secured by estrogens and androgens.

In this account, only the surface of the contribution of endocrine organs to fetal internal environment has been touched. That the endocrine organs profoundly modify behavior in postnatal life is clear, but the beginnings of their activity and hence of their effects upon prenatal behavior are still so uncertain that more adequate treatment here of an intensely interesting field has seemed neither necessary nor wise.

* * * * * *

Evidence so far gathered appears to indicate that the behavior of vertebrate animals, including man, has its genesis in the early exteroceptive responses exhibited during embryonic, larval, or fetal life. It would seem probable that there is a basic similarity in the succession of responses which may be elicited from vertebrate organisms in response to external stimulation. However, it is evident that each class of vertebrates, perhaps each order, genus, and species, exhibits characteristics in the development of behavior which belong to that subdivision of animals alone. Nevertheless, each form of activity shown by any fetal organism is a step in normal development, hence a step in preparation for postnatal behavioral capabilities. Furthermore, there is a tendency for voluntary acts, where and when they appear, to develop in a sequence based upon the earlier reflexogenic sequence of prenatal life. This is particularly well demonstrated in the case of human behavior. The frontiers of research in the development of fetal activity are by no means closed. Final proof of the exact nature of many steps in the development of prenatal activity in many forms is yet to come, but it would appear that a reasonably sound foundation has been laid by the work of many investigators, upon which future studies in the field may rest.

Notes

1. See C. Judson Herrick's *George Ellett Coghill*, 1949, a mine of information regarding the man and his work.

2. In this connection, see Herrick, 1949, p. 238, note 42.

3. R. G. Harrison's staging of *Amblystoma* embryos on the basis of morphological characteristics has, unfortunately, never been published as a whole, but photographs of Miss Lisbeth Krause's beautiful drawings of each stage have been widely distributed to investigators. Harrison's stages differ from Coghill's, as the latter were based on physiological criteria.

4. Dr. Coghill has objected (1940, p. 44, note) to the acceptance of Swenson's thesis as a published source, inasmuch as it was never approved in toto for publication, some changes being desirable. However, as it is the only present source of Swenson's earlier views, it is here used with the qualification just stated.

5. For another, and excellent, review of vertebrate behavioral development, the reader is referred to Carmichael (1946).

6. The term "case" is used to denote each pregnancy terminated spontaneously or by operation, regardless of whether the "case" furnished one or more fetuses.

7. The writer wishes to express to Dr. Tryphena Humphrey his thanks for permission to use in the third Porter Lecture presented at Kansas City on March 13, 1951, lantern slides of her diagrams of the caudal extent of the divisions of the trigeminal nerve and of the connections found to form the reflex arc in the earliest responses of human embryos to exteroceptive stimulation in the perioral region. These diagrams were presented by Dr. Humphrey (1951) at the session of the American Association of Anatomists in Detroit on March 22, and some will be published in her article (1952a) in the *Journal of Comparative Neurology*. One, hitherto unpublished, is here presented as figure 5.

Acknowledgments

The writer takes pleasure in acknowledging with thanks permission to make quotations or to reproduce illustrations from published books or journals owned by the following:

To the Wistar Institute of Anatomy and Biology, Philadelphia, for excerpts from the *Journal of Cellular and Comparative Physiology*, the *Journal of Experimental Zoology* and the *Journal of Comparative Neurology*, including figures 4 and 6, tables 1, 2, and 4, and use of the Swenson-Coghill film of *Amblystoma*, and to the authors, Drs. Angulo, Barron, Humphrey, Sawyer, and Windle; to the University of Chicago Press, Chicago, for quotations from *George Ellett Coghill* by C. Judson Herrick, 1949, and for excerpts from *Physiological Zoology*, and to the authors, Drs. Herrick and Windle; to The Journal Press, Provincetown, Massachusetts, for quotations from *Genetic Psychology Monographs*, including table 3, and to the authors, Drs. Carmichael and Coronios; to the Cambridge University Press, Cambridge, England, for excerpts from the *Journal of Physiology* and to the author, Dr. Windle; and to the Yale University Press for a quotation from *Integrative Action of the Nervous System* by C. S. Sherrington, 1906, and to Sir Charles Sherrington, the author.

It is also a pleasure to acknowledge my debt to my colleagues, Drs. Tryphena Humphrey and John C. Donaldson, to Dr. Donald H. Barron, and to my wife, Helen Ferris Hooker, for their kindness in criticizing and correcting the manuscript at various stages of its completion, to Dr. Donaldson for his photographic assistance with the illustrative material, and to Dr. Humphrey for the use of figure 5, hitherto unpublished.

This book owes much to the wise counsel of Mr. Clyde K. Hyder, of the University of Kansas Press. His keen editorial eye and his knowledge of book production have been of great help to the author, who is deeply grateful.

Reference List

AHLFELD, F., 1905, Die intrauterine Tätigkeit der Thorax- und Zwerchfelmuskeln. Mon. f. Geb. u. Gynäk., *21:* 143-163.

ANGULO (Y GONZALEZ), ARMANDO W., 1927, The motor nuclei in the cervical cord of the albino rat at birth. J. Comp. Neur., *43:* 115-142.

———, 1929, Is myelinogeny an absolute index of behavioral capacity? J. Comp. Neur., *48:* 459-464.

———, 1930*a*, Neurological interpretation of fetal behavior: The progressive increase of muscular activity in albino-rat fetuses. Anat. Rec., *45:* 254.

———, 1930*b*, Endogenous stimulation of albino rat fetuses. Proc. Soc. Exp. Biol. and Med., *27:* 579.

———, 1932*a*, The prenatal growth of the albino rat. Anat. Rec., *52:* 117-138.

———, 1932*b*, The prenatal development of behavior in the albino rat. J. Comp. Neur., *55:* 395-442.

———, 1933, Development of somatic activity in the albino rat fetuses. Proc. Soc. Exp. Biol. and Med., *31:* 111-112.

———, 1935, Further studies upon development of somatic activity in albino rat fetuses. Proc. Soc. Exp. Biol. and Med., *32:* 621-622.

———, 1936, The neuro-mechanism of the trunk limb component of the total behavior pattern. Anat. Rec., *64,* Suppl. No. 3: 2-3.

———, 1939, Histogenesis of the monopolar neuroblast and the ventral longitudinal path in the albino rat. J. Comp. Neur., *71:* 325-360.

———, 1951a, A comparison of the growth and differentiation of the trigeminal ganglia with the ganglia of the cervical region in albino rat embryos. Anat. Rec., *109:* 391.

———, 1951*b*, A comparison of the growth and differentiation of the trigeminal ganglia with the cervical spinal ganglia in albino rat embryos. J. Comp. Neur., *95:* 53-71.

AVERY, GEORGE T., 1928, Responses of foetal guinea pigs prematurely delivered. Genet. Psychol. Monogr., *3:* 245-331.

BAER, KARL E. VON, 1828, Ueber Entwicklungsgeschichte der Thiere. 2 vols., Königsberg. (Cited from Preyer, 1885.)

BALFOUR, FRANCIS M., 1874, A preliminary account of the development of the elasmobranch fishes. Mem. Edit. Works of F. M. Balfour, *1:* 60-112, 1885.

———, 1878, A monograph on the development of the elasmobranch fishes. Mem. Edit. Works of F. M. Balfour, *1*: 203-520, 1885.

BALL, ERIC G., 1952, Oxidations and reductions in the brain tissue. Biological Aspects of Mental Health and Disease, Chap. 6, pp. 74-82 (Milbank Memor. Fund Symposium, Nov. 13-16, 1950). Hoeber, New York.

BARCROFT, JOSEPH, 1939, The intra-uterine development of respiratory effort. Brit. Med. J., Nov. 18, 1939: 986-987.

———, 1947, Researches in pre-natal life. Chas. C. Thomas, Springfield, Ill.

BARCROFT, JOSEPH, AND D. H. BARRON, 1936, The genesis of respiratory movements in the foetus of the sheep. J. Physiol., 88: 56-61.

———, 1937, Movements in midfoetal life in the sheep embryo. J. Physiol., *91*: 329-351.

———, 1939a, Movement in the mammalian foetus. Ergebn. d. Physiol., biol. Chem. u. exper. Pharmacol., *42*: 107-152.

———, 1939b, The development of behavior in foetal sheep. J. Comp. Neur., 70: 477-502.

BARCROFT, J., D. H. BARRON AND W. F. WINDLE, 1936, Some observations on genesis of somatic movements in sheep embryos. J. Physiol., *87*: 73-78.

BARRON, DONALD H., 1941, The functional development of some mammalian neuromuscular mechanisms. Biol. Rev., *16*: 1-33.

———, 1944, The early development of the sensory and internuncial cells in the spinal cord of the sheep. J. Comp. Neur., *81*: 193-225.

———, 1946, The oxygen pressure gradient between the maternal and fetal blood in pregnant sheep. Yale J. Biol. and Med., 19: 23-27.

———, 1950, Genetic neurology and the behavior problem. Genetic Neurology, ed. by P. Weiss: 223-231, Univ. of Chicago Press, Chicago.

———, 1951, Placental morphology and fetal respiration. Science, *114*: 477.

BECKER, R. F., W. F. WINDLE, E. E. BARTH, AND M. D. SCHULZ, 1940, Fetal swallowing, gastro-intestinal activity and defecation in utero. Surg., Gyn. and Obst., 70: 603-614.

BEGUELIN, 1757, Abhandlung von der kunstliche geöffnete Eier beim Lampenfeur auszubrüten. Hamburg. Mag. o. d. gesam. Schrift a. d. Naturforsch. u. d. angen. Wissen. überh., *19*: 118-156. (Cited from Preyer, 1885.)

BERSOT, H., 1920-1, Développment réactionnel et réflexe plantaire du bébé né avant terme à celui de deux ans. Schweiz. Arch. f. Neurol. u. Psychiatr., 7: 212-231; 8: 47-74.

Boell, Edward J., and S. C. Shen, 1950, Development of cholinesterase in the central nervous system of Amblystoma punctatum. J. Exp. Zool., 113: 583-600.

Bolaffio, M., and G. Artom, 1924, Richerche sulla fisiologia del sistema nervosa del feto umano. Arch. d. Scienze biol., 5: 457-487.

Boyd, Edith, 1941, Outline of physical growth and development. Burgess, Minneapolis.

Bregmann, E., 1892, Über experimentelle aufsteigende Degeneration motorischer und sensibler Hirnnerven. Arb. a. d. Inst. f. Anat. u. Physiol. d. C.n.s. a.d. Wiener Univ., 1: 73-97.

Bremer, John L., 1935, Postnatal development of alveoli in the mammalian lung in relation to the problem of the alveolar phagocyte. Carnegie Contrib. to Embryol., 25: 83-110.

Bridgman, C. S., and L. Carmichael, 1935, An experimental study of the onset of behavior in the fetal guinea-pig. J. Genet. Psychol., 47: 247-267.

Brinley, Floyd J., 1951, Studies on the effect of curare on spontaneous muscular activity in fish embryos. Physiol. Zool., 24: 186-195.

Brooks, C. McC., and J. E. Eccles, 1947, A study of the effects of anesthesia and asphyxia on the mono-synaptic pathway through the spinal cord. J. Neurophysiol., 10: 349-360.

Cajal, Santiago R., 1906, Génesis de las fibras nerviosas del embrión y observaciones contrarias a la teoría catenaria. Trabajos, Madrid, 4: 227-294.

Cannon, Walter B., and I. R. Burket, 1913, The endurance of anemia by nerve cells in the myenteric plexus. Am. J. Physiol., 32: 347-357.

Carlson, A. J., and F. M. Drennan, 1911, The control of pancreatic diabetes in pregnancy by the passage of the internal secretions of the pancreas of the fetus to the blood of the mother. Am. J. Physiol., 28: 391-395.

Carmichael, Leonard, 1934, An experimental study in the prenatal guinea-pig of the origin and development of reflexes and patterns of behavior in relation to the stimulation of specific receptor areas during the period of active fetal life. Genet. Psychol. Monogr., 16: 337-491.

———, 1946, The onset and early development of behavior. Chap. 2, Manual of Child Devel., ed. by L. Carmichael: 43-166. Wiley, New York.

Clark, Eleanor L., and E. R. Clark, 1914, On the early pulsations of the posterior lymph hearts in chick embryos: Their relation to the body movements. J. Exp. Zool., *17*: 373-394.

Clark, Sam L., 1947, Ranson's The anatomy of the nervous system. 8th Ed. W. B. Saunders, Philadelphia.

Coghill, George E., 1902, The cranial nerves of Amblystoma tigrinum. J. Comp. Neur., *12*: 205-289.

———, 1909, The reaction to tactile stimuli and the development of the swimming movement in embryos of Diemyctylus torosus Eschscholtz. J. Comp. Neur., *19*: 83-105.

———, 1914-1936, Correlated anatomical and physiological studies of the growth of the nervous system of Amphibia. J. Comp. Neur., I, *24*: 161-233 (1914); II, *26*: 247-340 (1916); III, *37*: 37-69 (1924*a*); IV, *37*: 71-120 (1924*b*); V, *40*: 47-94 (1926a); VI, *41*: 95-152 (1926*b*); VII, *42*: 1-16 (1926c); VIII, *45*: 227-247 (1928); IX, *51*: 311-375 (1930*a*); X, *53*: 147-168 (1931), XI, *57*: 327-358 (1933a); XII, *64*: 135-167 (1936).

———, 1929, Anatomy and the problem of behavior. Cambridge Univ. Press, Cambridge, England.

———, 1930*b*, Anatomical growth of the nervous system in relation to behavior. Proc. Conf. on Adolesc., Publ. as: Physical and mental adolescent growth: 106-110.

———1930c, The structural basis of the integration of behavior. Proc. Nat. Acad. Sci., *16*: 637-643.

———, 1933*b*, Somatic myogenic action in embryos of Fundulus heteroclitus. Proc. Soc. Exp. Biol. and Med., *31*: 62-64.

———, 1940, Early embryonic somatic movements in birds and in mammals other than man. Monogr. Soc. Res. Child Devel., *5*: No. 2.

Coronios, J. D., 1933, Development of behavior in the fetal cat. Genet. Psychol. Monogr., *14*: 283-386.

Cuthbert, F. G., A. C. Ivy, B. L. Isaacs, and J. Gray, 1940, The relation of pregnancy and lactation to extirpation diabetes in the dog. Am. J. Physiol., *115*: 480-496.

Davis, M. Edward, and Edith L. Potter, 1946, Intrauterine respiration of the human fetus. J. A. M. A., *131*: 1194-1201.

Donaldson, John C., and Tryphena Humphrey, 1949, Cells with argentophilic granules in the embryonic human pancreas. Anat. Rec., *103*: 532-533.

Emmert, A. G. F., and Hochstetter, 1811, Die Entwicklung der Eidechsen in ihren Eiern. Arch. f. d. Physiol., *10*: 86, 95, 100-104, 376. (Cited from Preyer, 1885.)

ERBKAM, 1837, Lebhafte Bewegung eines viermonatlichen Fötus. Neue Zeitschr. f. Geburtsk., 5: 324-326.

FERNER, HELMUT, 1938, Über die Entwicklung der Langerhansschen Inseln nach der Geburt und die Bedeutung der versilberbaren Zellen im Pankreas des Menschen. Zeitsch. f. mikr.-anat. Forschung, 44: 451-488.

FITZGERALD, JAMES E., AND W. F. WINDLE, 1942, Some observations on early human fetal activity. J. Comp. Neur., 76: 159-167.

GESELL, ARNOLD, WITH C. S. AMATRUDA, 1945, The embryology of behavior. Harper, New York.

GOSS, C. M., 1940, First contractions of the heart without cytological differentiation. Anat. Rec., 76: 19-27.

GROSSER, OTTO, 1927, Frühentwicklung, Eihautbildung, und Placentation. Bergmann, Munich.

GUTHMANN, H., AND W. MAY, 1930, Gibt es intrauterine Nierensekretion? Arch. f. Gynäk., *141*: 450-459.

HALVERSON, H. M., 1937, Studies of the grasping responses of early infancy. J. Genet. Psychol., 51: 371-449.

———, 1943, The development of prehension in infants. Child Devel. and Behavior, ed. by Barker, Kounin, and Wright, Chap. 4: 49-65. McGraw-Hill, New York.

HARREVELD, A. VAN, 1944, Survival of reflex contractions and inhibition during cord asphyxia. Am. J. Physiol., *141*: 97-101.

HARRISON, ROSS G., 1904, An experimental study of the relation of the nervous system to the developing musculature in the embryo of the frog. Am. J. Anat., 3: 197-220.

———, 1910, The outgrowth of the nerve fiber as a mode of protoplasmic movement. J. Exp. Zool., 9: 787-848.

HARVEY, WILLIAM, 1651, Exercitationes de generatione animalium. Pulleyn, London. (See Meyer, 1936.)

HELD, HANS, 1909, Die Entwicklung des Nervengewebes bei den Wirbeltieren. Barth, Leipzig.

HENSEN, V., 1903, Die Entwicklungsmechanik der Nervenbahnen im Embryo der Säugetiere. Kiel.

HERRICK, C. JUDSON, 1949, George Ellett Coghill, Naturalist and Philosopher. Univ. of Chicago Press, Chicago, Ill.

HERRICK, C. JUDSON, AND G. E. COGHILL, 1915, The development of reflex mechanisms in Amblystoma. J. Comp. Neur., 25: 65-85.

HEWER, EVELYN E., 1938, Textbook of histology for medical students. Mosby, St. Louis.

HIMWICH, HAROLD E., 1951, Brain metabolism and cerebral disorders. Williams and Wilkins, Baltimore.

HIS, WILHELM, 1887, Die Entwicklung der ersten Nervenbahnen beim menschlichen Embryo. Arch. f. Anat. u. Physiol., Anat. Abt., Jahrg. 1887, 368-378.

HOME, EVERARD, 1822, On the changes the egg undergoes during incubation. Philos. Trans. Roy. Soc. Lond., *2*: 339-356.

HOOKER, DAVENPORT, 1936, Early fetal activity in mammals. Yale J. Biol. and Med., *8*: 579-602.

———, 1938, The origin of the grasping movement in man. Proc. Am. Philos. Soc., *79*: 597-606.

———, 1939, Fetal behavior. Res. Publ. Assn. Res. Nerv. and Ment. Dis., *19*: 237-243.

———, 1942, Fetal reflexes and instinctual processes. Psychosom. Med., *4*: 199-205.

———, 1943, Reflex activities in the human fetus. Child Behav. and Devel., ed. by Barker, Kounin and Wright, Chap. 2: 17-28. McGraw-Hill, New York.

———, 1944, The origin of overt behavior. Univ. of Mich. Press, Ann Arbor.

HOUSSAY, BERNARDO A., 1951, Human physiology. McGraw-Hill Book Co., Inc., New York.

HULTQUIST, GÖSTA T., 1946, On the occurrence of s. c. silver cells in islet tumors and in the pancreas in cases of islet tumors. Gastroenterologia, *71*: 193-209.

HUMPHREY, TRYPHENA, 1944, Primitive neurons in the embryonic human central nervous system. J. Comp. Neur., *81*: 1-45.

———, 1951, The caudal extent of the descending root of the trigeminal nerve during the period of early human fetal activity (8 to 8.5 weeks of menstrual age). Anat. Rec., *109*: 306-307.

———, 1952*a*, The spinal tract of the trigeminal nerve in human embryos between 7½ and 8½ weeks of menstrual age and in relation to fetal behavior. J. Comp. Neur., *96*: 1-67.

———, 1952*b*, The relation of oxygen deprivation to fetal reflex arcs and the development of fetal behavior. J. Psychol., *34* (in press).

HUMPHREY, TRYPHENA, AND J. C. DONALDSON, 1949, Argentophile cells in the early embryonic human pancreas. Anat. Rec., *103*: 572.

KATO, GENICHI, 1934, The microphysiology of nerve. Mazuren, Tokyo, pp. 139.

KERR, J. GRAHAM, 1910, The development of the peripheral nerves of vertebrates. Proc. Roy. Phys. Soc. Edinburgh, *18*: 11-20.

KRABBE, KNUD, 1912, Les réflexes chez le foetus. Rev. Neurol., *24*: 434-435.

KUO, ZING Y. 1932-1938, Ontogeny of embryonic behavior in birds. I, J. Exp. Zool., *61*: 395-430 (1932*a*); II, J. Exp. Zool., *62*: 453-487 (1932*b*); III, J. Comp. Psychol., *13*: 245-271 (1932*c*); IV, J. Comp. Psychol., *14*: 109-122 (1932*d*); V, Psychol. Rev., *39*: 499-515 (1932*e*); VI, J. Comp. Psychol., *16*: 379-384 (1933); X (wtih T. C. SHEN), J. Comp. Psychol., *21*: 87-93 (1936); XI (with T. C. SHEN), J. Comp. Psychol., *24*: 49-58 (1937); XII, Am. J. Psychol., *51*: 361-379 (1938).

———, 1939, Studies on the physiology of the embryonic nervous system. IV. Development of acetylcholine in the chick embryo. J. Neurophysiol., *2*: 488-493.

KUTNER, R., AND F. KRAMER, 1907, Sensibilitätsstörungen bei acuten und chronischen Bulbärerkrankungen. Arch. f. Psychiatr., *42*: 1002-1006.

LANE, H. H., 1917, The correlation between structure and function in the development of the special senses of the white rat. Univ. Okla. Bull., No. 140 (Univ. Studies No. 8): 1-88.

LANGREDER, WILHELM, 1949, Welche Fötalreflexe haben eine intrauterine Aufgabe. Deutsch. Med. Wochenschr., *74*: 661-667.

LE GROS CLARK, W. E., 1945, The tissues of the body. 2nd Edit. Clarendon Press, Oxford.

LIESCH, E., 1946, La motilità riflessa durante lo sviluppo fetale nell' uomo. Boll. Soc. Ital. Biol. Sper., *22*: 831-833.

LILLIE, FRANK R., 1917, The freemartin: a study of the action of sex hormones in the foetal life of cattle. J. Exp. Zool., *23*: 371-452.

LLOYD, DAVID P. C., 1943a, Reflex action in relation to pattern and peripheral source of afferent stimulation. J. Neurophysiol., *6*: 111-119.

———, 1943b, Conduction and synaptic transmission of reflex response to stretch in spinal cats. J. Neurophysiol., *6*: 317-326.

MATTHEWS, S. A., AND S. R. DETWILER, 1926, The reactions of Amblystoma embryos following prolonged treatment with chloretone. J. Exp. Zool., *45*: 279-292.

MEYER, ARTHUR W., 1936, An analysis of the De Generatione Animalium of William Harvey. Stanford Univ. Press.

MINKOWSKI, M. 1920*a*, Réflexes et mouvements de la tête, du tronc et des extrémités du foetus humain, pendant la première moitie de la grossesse. C. R. d. l. Soc. Biol., *83*: 1202-1204.

———, 1920*b*, Movimientos y reflejos del feto humano durante la primera mitad del emberazo. Trabajos, Madrid, *18*: 269-273.

———, 1920*c*, Über Bewegungen und Reflexe des menschlichen Foetus während der ersten Hälfte seiner Entwicklung. Schweiz. Arch. f. Neurol. u. Psychiatr., 7: 148-151.

———, 1921, Sur les mouvements, les réflexes et les réactions musculaires du foetus humain de 2 à 5 mois et leurs relations avec le système nerveux foetal. Revue Neurol., 37: 1105-1118, 1235-1250.

———, 1922, Über frühzeitige Bewegungen, Reflexe und muskuläre Reaktionen beim menschlichen Foetus und ihre Beziehungen zum foetalen Nerven und Muskelsystem. Schweiz. med. Wochenschr., 3: 721-724, 751-755.

———, 1923, Zur Entwicklungsgeschichte, Lokalisation und Klinik des Fussohlenreflexes. Schweiz. Arch. f. Neurol. u. Psychiatr., 13: 475-514.

———, 1925, Zum gegenwärtigen Stand der Lehre von den Reflexen. Neurol. u. Psychiatr. Abhandl., Schweizer Archiv. f. Neurol. u. Psychiatr., *1*: 1-61.

———, 1924-5, Zum gegenwärtigen Stand der Lehre von der Reflexen. (in entwicklungsgeschichtlicher und anatomish-physiologischer Beziehung) Schweiz. Arch. f. Neurol. u. Psychiatr., *15*: 239-259; *16*: 133-152, 266-284.

———, 1926, Sur les modalités et la localisation du réflexe plantaire au cours de son évolution du foetus à l'adulte. Congres d. med. alién. et neurol. de France et d. pays d. lang. franc., 30: 301-308.

———, 1927, Über du elektrische Erregbarkeit der foetalen Muskulatur. Schweiz. Arch. f. Neurol. u. Psychiat., 22: 64-72.

———, 1928, Neurobiologische Studien am menschlichen Foetus. Handbuch d. biol. Arbeitsmethoden. E. Abderhalden, Abt. V, Teil 5 B, Heft 5, Ser. Nr. 253: 511-618.

———, 1936, Cervical and labyrinthine reflexes in the human fetus. (Original in Russian.) Symp. on problems of nervous physiology and behavior, in honor of Prof. J. S. Beritoff. USSR Acad. Sci., Georgian Br.: 249-258.

———, 1946, Sur le développement et la localisation des fonctions nerveuses, surtout des mouvements et des réflexes, chez le foetus et le nouveau-né. Atti d. Congr. Italo-Svizzero d. Neuropsicol. Infantile: 35-57.

———, 1946, Sur l' évolution anatomo-physiologique des fonctions cérébrales chez le nourisson et le petit enfant. Atti d. Congr. Italo-Svizz. d. Neuropsicol. Infantile: 59-80.

———, 1947, Sur le début d'une évolution biopsychique chez le foetus. C. R. d. Congr. d. Med. Alién. et Neurol., 45th session: 1-10.

Moore, Carl R., 1947, Embryonic sex hormones and sexual differentiation. Chas. C. Thomas, Springfield, Ill.

———, 1950, The role of the fetal endocrine glands in development. J. Clin. Endocrin., *10*: 942-985.

Mossman, Harland W., 1937, Comparative morphogenesis of the fetal membranes and accessory uterine structures. Carnegie Contrib. to Embryol., *26*: 129-246.

Needham, Joseph, 1931, Chemical Embryology. Cambridge Univ. Press, 3 vols.

Orr, Douglas W., and W. F. Windle, 1934, The development of behavior in chick embryos: the appearance of somatic movements. J. Comp. Neur., *60*: 271-285.

Pankratz, D. S., 1931, A preliminary report on the fetal movements in the rabbit. Anat. Rec., *48*: Suppl., 58-59.

Paton, Stewart, 1905, The reactions of the vertebrate embryo to stimulation and the associated changes in the nervous system. Mitt. a. d. zool. Stat. zu Neapel, *18*: 535-581.

———, 1911, The reactions of the vertebrate embryo and associated changes in the nervous system. Second paper. J. Comp. Neur., *21*: 345-373.

Pflüger, E. F. W., 1877, Die Lebenszähigkeit des menschlichen Foetus. Arch. f. d. ges. Physiol., *14*: 628-629.

Preyer, Wilhelm, 1822, Die Seele des Kindes, Beobachten über die geistige Entwicklung des Menschen in den ersten Lebensjahren. Fernau, Leipzig.

———, 1885, Specielle Physiologie des Embryo. Grieben, Leipzig.

Ranson, S. Walter, 1943, The anatomy of the nervous system. 7th ed. W. B. Saunders, Philadelphia.

Rawitz, Bernhard, 1879, Lebenszähigkeit des Embryo. Arch f. Physiol., Suppl. Bd: 69-71.

Reifferscheid, K., 1911, Ueber intrauterine Atembewegungen des Foetus. Arch. f. d. ges Physiol., *140*: 1-16.

Remak, R., 1854, Die Zusammenziehung des Amnions. Arch. f. Anat., Physiol., u. wiss. Med.: 369-373. (Cited from Preyer, 1885.)

Rosenfeld, Morris, and F. F. Snyder, 1936, Foetal respiration in the rabbit. Proc. Soc. Exp. Biol. and Med., *33*: 576-578.

Sawyer, Charles H., 1934a, Cholinesterase and the behavior problem in Amblystoma. I. The relationship between the development of the enzyme and early motility. II. The effects of inhibiting cholinesterase. J. Exp. Zool., *92*: 1-29.

———, 1943b, Cholinesterase and the behavior problem in Amblystoma. III. The distribution of cholinesterase in nerve and muscle throughout development. IV. Cholinesterase in nerveless muscle. J. Exp. Zool., *94*: 1-31.

———, 1944, Nature of the early somatic movements in Fundulus heteroclitus. J. Cell. and Comp. Physiol., *24*: 71-84.

Schlesinger, H., 1895, Die Syringomyélie. Deutlicke, Leipzig.

Sherrington, Charles S., 1906, The integrative action of the nervous system. Yale Univ. Press, New Haven, Conn.

———, 1910, Notes on the scratch reflex of the cat. Q. J. Exp. Physiol., *3*: 213-220.

Sjöqvist, O., 1938, Studies on pain conduction in the trigeminal nerve. Acta Psychiatr. et Neurol., Suppl. No. 17: 1-139.

Smith, Karl U., and Robert S. Daniel, 1946, Observations of behavioral development in the loggerhead turtle (Caretta caretta). Science, *104*: 154-155.

Smyth, G. E., 1939, The systemization and central connections of the spinal tract and nucleus of the trigeminal nerve. A clinical and pathological study. Brain, 62: 41-87.

Snyder, Franklin F., and M. Rosenfeld, 1937a, Direct observation of intrauterine respiratory movements of the fetus and the role of carbon dioxide and oxygen in their regulation. Am. J. Physiol., *119*: 153-166.

———, 1937*b*, Breathing of amniotic fluid as a normal function of fetal respiration. Proc. Soc. Exp. Biol. and Med., *36*: 45-46.

———, 1937c, Intrauterine respiratory movements of the human fetus. J. A. M. A., *108*: 1946-1948.

Sölder, F. von, 1899, Der segementale Begrenzungstypus bei Hautanaesthesien am Kopfe, insbesondere in Fälle von Syringomyelie. Jahrb. f. Psychiatr. u. Neurol., 18: 458-478.

Spiller, W. G., 1908, The symptom-complex of occlusion of the posterior inferior cerebellar artery: two cases with necropsy. J. Nerv. and Ment. Dis., 35: 365-387.

Steele, A. G., and W. F. Windle, 1939, Some correlations between respiratory movements and blood gasses in cat foetuses. J. Physiol., 94: 531-538.

———, 1939, The oxygen and carbon dioxide content of the blood of normal and pregnant decerebrate cats. J. Physiol., *94*: 525-530.

Stopford, John S. B., 1924, The function of the spinal nucleus of the trigeminal nerve. J. Anat., 59: 120-128.

Strassman, P., 1903, Das Leben vor der Geburt. Samml. Klin. Vortr., no. 353 (Gynäk. No. 132): 947-968.

STRAUS, WILLIAM L., JR., AND G. WEDDELL, 1940, Nature of the first visible contractions of the forelimb musculature in rat fetuses. J. Neurophysiol., 3: 358-369.

STREETER, GEORGE L., 1920, Weight, sitting height, head size, foot length and menstrual age of the human embryo. Carnegie Contrib. to Embryol., *11*: 143-170.

SWENSON, ENGELBREKT A., 1926, The development of movement of the albino rat before birth. Thesis, Univ. Kansas (unpublished).

———, 1928, The simple movements of the trunk of the albino rat. Anat. Rec., 38: 31.

———, 1929, The active simple movements of the albino rat fetus: the order of their appearance, their qualities, and their significance. Anat. Rec., *42*: 40.

TILNEY, FREDERICK, 1933, Behavior in its relation to the development of the brain. II. Bull. Neur. Inst. N. Y., 3: 252-358.

TILNEY, FREDERICK, AND L. S. KUBIE, 1931, Behavior in its relation to the development of the brain. I. Bull. Neur. Inst. N. Y., *1*: 229-313.

TRACY, HENRY C., 1925, Relation of CO_2 to spontaneous movements in the larvae of Opsanus tau. Biol. Bull., 48: 408-411.

———,1926, The development of motility and behavior reactions in the toadfish (Opsanus tau). J. Comp. Neur., 40: 253-369.

TUGE, HIDEOMI, 1931, Early behavior of the embryos of the turtle, Terrapene carolina (L.). Proc. Soc. Exp. Biol. and Med., 29: 52-53.

———, 1934, Early behavior of the embryos of carrier-pigeons. Proc. Soc. Exp. Biol. and Med., *31*: 462-463.

———, 1937, The development of behavior in avian embryos. J. Comp. Neur., 66: 157-179.

VALENCIENNES, 1841, Observations faites pendant l'incubation d'une femelle du Python bivittatus. Annal. d. Sci. Natur., *16*: 65-72. (Cited from Preyer, 1885.)

VALKENBURG, C. T. VAN, 1911, Zur Kenntnis der Radix spinalis nervi trigemini. Monatschr. f. Psychiatr. u. Neurol., 29: 407-437.

VULPIAN, A., 1857, La physiologie de l'amnios et d' allantoide chez les oiseaux. Mém. l. à l. Soc. de Biol., Ser. 2, 4: 269-278. (Cited from Preyer, 1885.)

WALLENBERG, ADOLF, 1896, Die secundäre Bahn des sensiblen Trigeminus. Anat. Anz., *12*: 95-110.

WANG, GING HSI, AND T. W. LU, 1940, Spontaneous activity of spinal tadpoles of frog and toad. Science, 92: 148.

———, 1941, Development of swimming and righting reflexes in frog (Rana guentheri): Effects thereon of transection of central nervous system before hatching. J. Neurophysiol., *4*: 137-146.

WEISS, PAUL, 1941*a* Autonomous versus reflexogenous activity of the central nervous system. Proc. Am. Philos. Soc., *84*: 53-64.

———, 1941*b*, Does sensory control play a constructive role in the development of motor co-ordination? Schweiz. med. Wochenschr., 71st year: 591-595.

———, 1941*c*, Self differentiation of the basic patterns of co-ordination. Psychol. Monogr., No. 88, *17*: 1-96.

WHITE, GERTRUDE M., 1915, The behavior of brook trout embryos from the time of hatching to the absorption of the yolk sac. J. Anim. Behav., *5*: 44-60.

WINDLE, WILLIAM F., 1930, The earliest fetal movements in the cat correlated with the neurofibrillar development of the spinal cord. Anat. Rec., *45*: 249.

———, 1931, The neurofibrillar structure of the spinal cord correlated with the appearance of early somatic movements. J. Comp. Neur., *53*: 71-113.

———, 1933, Neurofibrillar development in the central nervous system of cat embryos between 8 and 12 mm. long. J. Comp. Neur., *58*: 643-723.

———, 1934*a*, Correlation between the development of spinal reflexes and reflex arcs in albino-rat embryos. Anat. Rec., *58*: Suppl. Am. Assn. Anat., 42.

———, 1934*b*, Correlation between the development of local reflexes and reflex arcs in the spinal cord of rat embryos. J. Comp. Neur., *59*: 487-505.

———, 1936, The genesis of somatic behaviour in mammalian embryos. J. Physiol., *87*: 31P-33P.

———, 1937, On the nature of the first forelimb movements of mammalian embryos. Proc. Soc. Exp. Biol. and Med., *36*: 640-642.

———, 1940, Physiology of the fetus. Saunders, Philadelphia.

———, 1944, Genesis of somatic motor function in mammalian embryos: a synthesizing article. Physiol. Zool., *17*: 247-260.

———, 1950*a*, Asphyxia neonatorum. Charles C. Thomas, Springfield, Ill.

———, 1950*b*, Reflexes of mammalian embryos and fetuses. Genetic Neurology, ed. by Paul Weiss, Univ. of Chicago Press: 214-222.

WINDLE, W. F., AND R. E. BAXTER, 1936, Development of reflex mechanisms in the spinal cord of albino rat embryos. Correlations between structure and function, and comparisons with the cat and the chick. J. Comp. Neur., 63: 189-209.

WINDLE, W. F., AND R. F. BECKER, 1940, Relation of anoxemia to early activity in the fetal nervous system. Arch. Neur. and Psych., 43: 90-101.

WINDLE, W. F., R. F. BECKER, E. E. BARTH, AND M. D. SCHULZ, 1939, Aspiration of amniotic fluid by the fetus. An experimental roentgenological study in the guinea pig. Surg., Gyn. and Obst., 69: 705-712.

WINDLE, W. F., R. F. BECKER, RUTH RHINES, AND ELIZABETH J. COWGILL, 1942, Effects of anoxia on trigeminal reflexes in cat fetuses. Physiol. Zool., 15: 375-382.

WINDLE, W. F., AND C. L. BISHOP, 1939, Prenatal intestinal movements in anoxia. Proc. Soc. Exp. Biol. and Med., 40: 2-4.

WINDLE, W. F., C. A. DRAGSTEDT, D. E. MURRAY AND R. R. GREENE, 1938, A note on the respiration-like movements of the human fetus. Surg., Gynec. and Obst., 66: 987-988.

WINDLE, W. F., AND M. W. FISH, 1923, The development of the vestibular righting reflex in the cat. J. Comp. Neur., 54: 85-96.

WINDLE, W. F., AND J. E. FITZGERALD, 1937, Development of the spinal reflex mechanism in human embryos. J. Comp. Neur., 67: 493-509.

WINDLE, W. F., AND A. M. GRIFFIN, 1931, Observations on embryonic and fetal movements of the cat. J. Comp. Neur., 52: 149-188.

WINDLE, W. F., W. L. MINEAR, M. F. AUSTIN, AND D. W. ORR, 1935, The origin and early development of somatic behavior in the albino rat. Physiol. Zool., 8: 156-185.

WINDLE, W. F., M. MONNIER AND A. G. STEELE, 1938, Fetal respiratory movements in the cat. Physiol. Zool., 11: 425-433.

WINDLE, W. F., J. E. O'DONNELL, AND F. E. GLASSHAGLE, 1933, The early development of spontaneous and reflex behavior in cat embryos and fetuses. Physiol. Zool., 6: 521-541.

WINDLE, W. F., AND D. W. ORR, 1934, The development of behavior in chick embryos: spinal cord structure correlated with early somatic motility. J. Comp. Neur., 60: 287-307.

WINDLE, W. F., D. W. ORR, AND W. L. MINEAR, 1934, The origin and development of reflexes in the cat during the third fetal week. Physiol. Zool., 7: 600-617.

WINDLE, W. F., AND A. G. STEELE, 1938, Reciprocal oxygen changes on both sides of placenta during uterine contraction and relaxation. Proc. Soc. Exper. Biol. and Med., 39: 246-248.

WINKLER, CORNELIS, 1921, Le système du nerf trijumeau. Opera Omnia, 7: 1-100.

WINTERSTEIN, H., 1914, Ueberleben eines menschlichen Fötus bei kunstliche Durchspülung. Deutsch. Physiol. Gesell., Zentralbl. f. Physiol., 28: 728.

WINTREBERT, P., 1920, La contraction rythmée aneurale des myotomes chez lez embryons de sélaciens. I. Observation de Scylliorhinus canicula L. Gill. Arch. de Zool. Exper. et Gen., *60*: 221-459.

WINTROBE, M. M., AND H. B. SHUMACKER, JR., 1936, Erythrocyte studies in the mammalian fetus and newborn. Am. J. Anat., 58: 313-328.

WISLOCKI, GEORGE B., 1920, Experimental studies on fetal absorption. Carnegie Contrib. to Embryol., *11*: 45-60.

WOYCIECHOWSKI, B., 1928, Rucky zarodka ludzkiego 42 mm. Polsk. Gazeta Lekarska, 7: 409-411.

YANASE, J., 1907, Beiträge zur Physiologie der peristaltischen Bewegungen des embryonalen Darmes. Arch. f. d. ges. Physiol., *117*: 345-383; *119*: 451-464.

YOUNGSTROM, KARL A., 1938, Studies on the developing behavior of Anura. J. Comp. Neur., *68*: 351-379.

———, 1941, Acetylocholine esterase concentration during the development of the human fetus. J. Neurophysiol., *4*: 473-477.

———, 1944, Intramedullary sensory type ganglion cells in the spinal cord of human embryos. J. Comp. Neur., *81*: 47-53.

ZUNTZ, NATHAN, 1877, Ueber die Respiration des Saügetierfoetus. Arch. f. d. ges. Physiol., *14*: 605-627.

Index of Names

(Italicized page numbers refer to items in the Reference List.)

Subject Index

(Italicized page references are to figures or tables on the pages cited.)